Just Life

Just Life

BIOETHICS AND
THE FUTURE OF
SEXUAL DIFFERENCE

Mary C. Rawlinson

Columbia University Press
New York

Columbia University Press
Publishers Since 1893
New York   Chichester, West Sussex
cup.columbia.edu
Copyright © 2016 Columbia University Press

Library of Congress Cataloging-in-Publication Data
Names: Rawlinson, Mary C.
Title: The right to life: bioethics and the future of sexual difference /
Mary C. Rawlinson.
Description: New York : Columbia University Press, [2016] |
Includes bibliographical references and index.
Identifiers: LCCN 2015018088 | ISBN 9780231171748 (cloth : alk. paper) |
ISBN 9780231171755 (pbk. : alk. paper) | ISBN 9780231541190 (e-book)
Subjects: LCSH: Feminist theory. | Bioethics.
Classification: LCC HQ1190. R39 2016 | DDC 305.4201—dc23
LC record available at http://lccn.loc.gov/2015018088

∞

Columbia University Press books are printed on permanent
and durable acid-free paper.

This book is printed on paper with recycled content.
Printed in the United States of America

Cover design: Jordan Wannemacher
Cover image: © The Trustees of the British Museum

References to websites (URLs) were accurate at the time of writing. Neither the
author nor Columbia University Press is responsible for URLs that may have
expired or changed since the manuscript was prepared.

To Alexander and the future
And in grateful memory of those who came before
and are no longer here
Guinevere Hornsby Rawlinson, Robert Moledis Rawlinson Jr.,
and Mary Louisa Hall Rawlinson

Contents

Preface

All the speculation about overcoming the natural in the universal forgets that nature is not *one*. . . . *The* universal has been thought as *one*, thought on the basis of *one*. But this *one* does not exist.

—LUCE IRIGARAY, "HUMAN NATURE IS TWO" (1996)

One thing I want to say to all who would dismiss my feminist criticisms of my culture, using my "westernization" as a whiplash, is that my mother's pain too has rustled among the pages of all those books I have read that partly constitute my "Westernization," and has crept into all the suitcases I have ever packed for my several exiles.

—UMA NARAYAN, "CONTESTING CULTURES" (1997)

An international feminism that is going to have any bite quickly gets involved in making normative recommendations that cross boundaries of culture, nation, religion, race, and class.

—MARTHA NUSSBAUM, *WOMEN AND HUMAN DEVELOPMENT* (2000)

A BAND OF frolicking girls at liberty. A mother who will not give up her daughter who is also a mother. A girl with a book. Might these be figures of the universal in human experience?

Philosophy seems to offer only two attitudes toward the universal. Either the philosopher commits to the task of articulating the universal forms and laws of experience under the regulative ideal of the One, as if human experience could be captured in a single narrative, or the philosopher criticizes the idea of the universal for this very commitment and, in exposing the exclusions that are required to install the supposedly generic subject of the one narrative, rejects the idea of the universal altogether.

Critical phenomenology starts from the idea that universality appears in multiplicity and difference. More than one narrative will be necessary to do justice to life. Women's experience (and there will be others) is just as much an opportunity for the appearance of the universal as is Man's. Critical phenomenology resists both abstract universalism and cultural relativism.

Critical phenomenology analyses the forms and laws of experience as determined by a history of power in order to open the opportunity for other narratives and figures of identity. More than an adjustment in the distribution of goods, justice requires new styles of life and new forms of association, reflecting, beyond the rights of Man, universals aimed at health and happiness, rather than the concentration of wealth and the proliferation of elite zones of security.

The infrastructures that support the subjection of women, the capitalization of their bodies, and the marginalization of women in public debate are transcultural and make transcultural critique necessary to critical phenomenology. The irreducibility of sexual difference makes solidarity possible.

Both Saudi Arabia and the United States embrace the rhetoric of rights, but tolerate, as if it were unremarkable, limitations on women's bodily sovereignty, their access to meaningful work, and their participation in decision making.

In Saudi Arabia, women are prohibited from driving. Women who violate the ban have been jailed and referred to "terrorist" courts. Women's mobility is restricted further by prescribed clothing and a lack of access to physical activity. In 2009, the kingdom closed all gyms for women. Saudi researchers have linked the current obesity epidemic among Saudi women to this imposed immobility. Women are largely confined to domestic space and domestic pursuits. Saudi women must have a male guardian and may not travel or conduct business without his assent. Saudi women cannot vote or take part in public decision making.[1] They lack mobility, independence, and voice. The women of Saudi Arabia are denied agency and mobility by their own culture, rather than by an occupying or enslaving power, and it is the critics of that subjection who are cast as a colonizing force, imposing "Western" concepts of liberty and freedom. The ability to make decisions for one's self, to move about and speak freely, to make one's own decisions about sexuality and reproduction, not to find one's body at the mercy of another: the assumption that these values are alien to Arab women not only serves security and wealth in the Anglo-European countries by leaving the relationship to Saudi Arabia undisturbed but also assumes that some classes of humanbodies are happy to surrender their agency, mobility, and bodies to others.

In the United States, a country supposedly founded on an inviolable commitment to religious freedom, the state continues to conspire with unconstitutional efforts to deny women access to basic health services such as contraception and pregnancy management. As for protecting the vulnerable: 85 percent of the victims of domestic violence in the United States are women. In a country founded on equality of opportunity, women make 20 percent less than men for comparable work. While African Americans and Hispanics are more than twice as likely to be poor as white Americans, women are poorer than men in all racial groups. A quarter of these women are mothers. In 2014, in this democracy, women held only 18.5 percent of the seats in the House of Representatives and 20 percent of the seats in the Senate. The fifteen-member Cabinet included three women, at Health and Human Services, the Interior, and Commerce. Four women served previously at Health and Human Services, Homeland Security, Labor, and State. No woman has ever served as president or vice president of the United States. While women comprise about half of graduating classes in law and medicine, they remain dramatically underrepresented among deans and department chairs. In 2014 twenty-five women serve as CEOs of a Fortune 500, only one in the top ten and only two in the top twenty-five. An additional twenty-eight women serve as CEOs of Fortune 501–one thousand companies. In every field of public life in the U.S., women have only very limited participation in decisions about the future.[2]

This double determination—the assignment of women to the body, to domesticity, and to sexuality, on the one hand, and the absence of women in positions of leadership in public life, on the other—is *all too familiar.* Women are dramatically underrepresented in political institutions *around the globe* and tend to be concentrated at lower ranks. The same absence of women in leadership afflicts business, academia, and other key civil and political institutions. Daily news reports present, *as if they were unremarkable*, photographs of leaders—political, financial, scientific, academic—that contain only or almost only men. Readers pass by them *as if they were unremarkable*, as if the absence of women in these councils of power were not a cause for urgency. While women's lack of voice and presence is taken for granted and globally so familiar as to be *unheard* and *unseen*, women continue to be almost silent and invisible in the councils that determine the future.

At the same time that women lack a voice in the collective enterprises that determine the community's future, women's bodies serve as battlegrounds for men. Armies use rape as a weapon of war: they will conquer not only the land but also the womb of the enemy, claiming all his generative space as a means of obliteration (Bangladesh, 1971 and Bosnia, 1992). In tribal areas of South Asia, elders decree that young girls should be raped as a means of resolving some disputes among men. A girl's brother insults, or appears to insult, a woman of a higher caste, so his sister is raped by the woman's male relatives in order to restore their family's "honor" (Jharkhand, India, 2014). Under tribalism women labor for men, but their bodies can also be used to settle debts or as the site of a man's violence against other men. The Serbian rapists acted against Bosnian *men*. The male relatives in Jharkhand are punishing *the brother* when they rape his sister.

Women in the United States may suffer fewer explicit restrictions than their Arab or South Asian sisters, but their bodies too remain contested sites in debates about high school dress codes or reproductive services. Men in positions of power continue to preempt women's decision making, arrogating to themselves the power to dispose of women's bodies in relation to men's own fears and needs.[3] Judicial and legislative decisions in the United States regarding reproductive freedom regularly reflect the way in which women's most intimate decisions are not entrusted to them, but made by councils led by and composed mostly of men.[4]

While women lack voice and frequently find themselves disposed of by others, their labor—often unpaid, regularly underpaid—remains essential to the community's economy. As Luce Irigaray has argued, allowing women to work in the public sphere, while they continue their traditional role as caregivers and managers of the domestic space, hardly promotes women's flourishing.[5] Women who enter into the paid workforce continue to shoulder the majority of domestic tasks. The difficulty of integrating these demands is left to individual women, but it calls for a new infrastructure other than the gender division of labor to support the nourishing of both work and family.[6]

Hegel argues that the entry of women into science, politics, and philosophy "puts the domains themselves in danger."[7] Most immediately, such a transgression of the difference between male and female work would threaten the bodies of the species by leaving them untended. If women were to leave the domain of living bodies for discursive pursuits as men have done, those bodies themselves would be endangered—unfed, unprotected, unnursed, *unmothered*. Caring for those in a dependent mode—the elderly or children or the infirm—becomes a social problem without the gender division of labor. On Anglo-European horizons, this problem has been addressed by a proliferation of nursing homes, child care centers, home health aides, and nannies, positions that tend to be staffed by women of limited socioeconomic means who are often racial minorities or immigrants. Their own families are deprived of their care and must make their own arrangements for children and other vulnerable members when these women are absent. The gender division of labor remains firmly in place.

Globally, most women who enter the paid labor force do so of necessity. They enter nonprofessional positions that do not lead to leadership, and they struggle constantly to resolve the demands of work and family. Those privileged women who enter leadership tracks in politics, science, and business also struggle to resolve intimate and professional commitments. Often the resolutions available to them exploit social inequity, as they become dependent on nannies and maids who can no longer take care of their own families. These struggles and the suffering associated with them call for new ways of thinking about work and a rethinking of the worker not as a unit cost of production but as a node in a network of relationships. The current dichotomy and lack of integration between work and family creates unhappiness and social inequity and calls urgently for change.

It also creates illness. In the United States the entry of women into the workforce in large numbers has resulted in a significant decrease in home cooking. The substitution of processed foods and industrially produced meals for home-cooked food has been linked directly to the obesity epidemic that currently affects 40 percent of American adults and 25 percent of American children.[8] Hegel rightly recognizes that there is labor to be done to sustain the community of mortal bodies. When this labor of sustaining the body is undone or done poorly, both the happiness and health of the community suffer. The gender division of labor is an efficient and well-installed solution to the problem of integrating multiple forms of generativity, work and family. This ancient solution will not be easy to dislodge. Currently, when a woman enters the discursive or professional domains of public life, she attempts the impossible, to graft the masculine model of professional life onto the figures of wife and mother. She manages the sleight of hand of the impossible, two full-time jobs, by enlisting the paid help of other women who must then find a way of managing their families . . . and so on. Lesbian and gay couples also confront this need to find solutions for integrating work and family.

Proclamations of *equal rights* have failed to ensure equity in pay or a fair share of leadership positions for women, because equality does not address the core problem of integrating work and family. In criticizing a politics of equality, Irigaray articulates the need for *gendered* rights that recognize the different capacities and destinies of the two sexes. Not only do women under the ideology of equality find themselves saddled with the labor of two genders, but the idea of equality also suggests that justice requires only the extension of the rights of Man, not the articulation of new rights and universals through the voices of women's experiences and the other experiences that are marginalized under Man's hegemony.

Beyond the material threat of untended bodies, the entry of women into the discursive domains, of science, politics, and philosophy, poses a *philosophical* danger: this transgression of the gender division of labor calls into question the status of Man as the generic figure of the human. If there are at least two, and more, narratives of experience, narratives that cannot be reduced one to the other, philosophy can no longer operate according to the logic of the One or the Same. If sexual difference is irreducible, then the universal cannot be thought as one. A woman is neither a special case, whose experience applies only to women, nor a mere variant or approximation of Man, whose experience is prefigured without remainder in his. There will be at least two, and more, narratives in which universals are displayed. There will be new narratives other than Man's, and new universals will appear in them.

CRITICAL PHENOMENOLOGY AND THE SPECIFICITY OF UNIVERSALS

Over the last four decades, many countries have remade their built environments to facilitate the participation of people with disabilities in public and professional life. Curbs have been made wheelchair accessible. Elevator buttons are labeled in braille. At the same time, research on the experience of people with disabilities has exposed the way in which *disability* is not a term limited to a particular population, the disabled; rather, disability, or dependency, is a universal feature of human experience. Every human being is dependent and disabled at times.[9] By remaking the built environment to facilitate the participation of disabled citizens, states imply a universal truth: the built environment ought to be determined, not by the interests of global capital, but by the conditions of human agency and engagement. The specificity of the experience of disability makes evident universal dimensions of human experience and the imperative in making public policy, and in particular in materializing public space, to prioritize life and generativity over wealth.

While Anglo-European legal systems focus almost exclusively on judgment and punishment, Acholi traditions of Northern Uganda offer an entirely different approach to crime, especially to crimes that have a communal scope. Valuing the restoration of social bonds over punishment, these traditions offer rituals of truth and reconciliation in which the confession of the crime is met with forgiveness. In the *Phenomenology of Spirit* Hegel advances the same figure of confession, forgiveness, and reconciliation as the drama in which a community of mutual recognition is realized, specifically identifying it with a suspension of the law. The specificity of the Acholi experience yields a universal truth: the judgment of the law will always need the supplement of confession, forgiveness, and reconciliation through which a community repairs itself and moves forward.

The idea of the universal does not imply that there is one set of forms and laws for human experience or one set of conditions for knowledge or justice. While physical science may be guided by the ideal of a unified theory, human experience gives rise to multiple narratives and to distinct forms of life, contiguous, distant, or overlapping. The philosophical endeavor to articulate universal conditions of experience that would be *the same for all* not only rests on the exclusion of women and others from the field of evidence, their differences rendered irrelevant or a perversion, but it also amounts to a childish attempt to touch the horizon of the sky. The philosopher, like other humans, will always be situated somewhere, not at the "outside of heaven," as in Socrates' beautiful myth. Philosophical activity happens somewhere and at some time and is confronted by specific opportunities and challenges. Concepts and laws prove their universality by successfully organizing and sustaining experience. Humans need narratives, concepts, and figures that create solidarities adequate to answer to the urgencies of identity and action in their place and time.

As Hegel argues, a form or law cannot be thought apart from its content. The universal would be an "empty husk" apart from its articulation as an infrastructure of life. The concept remains unthought and a mere abstraction unless its vivacity in the sensuous is inscribed within it. The specificity of its genealogy will always mark it, even as it transcends its own climate through transplantation into other landscapes.

Multiple universals coexist in an open phenomenological space. What I learn from the experience of disability need not be related to what I learn from the Acholi by a mutual reduction to a set of abstract concepts and principles. Ethical thinking requires transcendence of one's own experience, not to an a-topia or no-place, but to *some* place. Thinking through disability makes the familiar built environment strange. By transcending my own experience to this specific place, I discover the universal principle of crafting the built environment to promote sustainable human activity and relationships, rather than to serve the accumulation of wealth. Thinking through the rituals of the Acholi or the experience of South Africa in its transition from apartheid, I discover the universal need to temper justice and punishment with a spirit of forgiveness as a condition for a communal future.

Transcendence requires more than the proclamation that I have "suspended the natural attitude," as if I could divest myself of my beliefs, prejudices, and hopes with the wave of a concept.[10] Husserl's eidetic variation appears to take place in a uniform, undifferentiated space unmarked by any play of forces. While classical phenomenology depends on the fiction of a generic subject and a search for the possibility conditions of experience *in general*, critical phenomenology marries the irreducibility of sexual difference to the genealogical analysis of the specific infrastructures of experience. Critique exposes both the erasure of sexual difference in thought and the specificity of the forms of life installed and sustained by it. Critical phenomenology labors to make visible not the "universal structures of all knowledge or of all possible moral action" but the specific narratives that define what can be thought, said, and done and by whom.[11] It takes nothing for granted: every claim to truth, every concept depends on forces, institutions, and identities that can be exposed in their historical specificity.

Critical phenomenology reveals both the irreducible historicity of experience and the plasticity of its forms. It links critique to the unheard possibilities of experience. The opening to new narratives depends on making the familiar strange. The possibility of imagining ourselves otherwise depends on coming to see that what appears "universal, necessary or obligatory" is marked by "singularity, contingency, and . . . arbitrary constraint."[12] This is an arduous and risky movement in which "one detaches oneself from what is accepted as true and seeks other rules."[13] Turning the familiar infrastructure of experience into a strange object may reveal the contingency of its necessary history. That the narrative and its rules might have been otherwise makes it possible to imagine that the infrastructures of experience might be otherwise. The moment of critique invites the articulation of new figures of life.

The invocation of "culture" to deflect criticism of the systematic subjection of women assumes that culture must always be respected, but a culture, apartheid South Africa or the Jim Crow South, does not deserve moral respect just because it exists. These cultures were ethically unsustainable and have ceased to exist.[14] This strategy of invoking respect for culture installs a false dichotomy between an abstract universalism and cultural relativism. The task of ethics is not to apply ready-to-hand abstract principles to empirical situations but to make injustice, suffering, and cruelty intolerable, so that they cease to exist. What is all too familiar must become strange.

BEYOND ABSTRACT RIGHT: REAL UNIVERSALS

Without sexual difference, there would be no life on earth . . . But let us return to nature. Restricting ourselves to humankind, let us state that neither man nor woman can manifest nor experience its totality. Each gender possesses or represents only one part of it. This reality is both very simple and quite foreign to our way of thinking.

—LUCE IRIGARAY, *I LOVE TO YOU* (1992)

From Hobbes to Hegel, Anglo-European philosophers pursue a method of abstraction by which the figure of the rational subject is installed as the norm or generic image of human experience. "All men reason alike."[15] This supposedly generic subject is produced through a serious of exclusions—women, children, savages, the infirm. By identifying human experience with the figure of Man or the rational subject, bioethics and philosophy impose a normative idea of what qualifies as human, a form of debate that plagues bioethics today. Even capabilities theory focuses on defining the essential properties of human flourishing in a way that opens it up to normative exclusions.[16]

At the same time, bioethics and philosophy meet moral urgencies, for the most part, by promulgating abstract rights and principles. Declaring the "equality of all human beings in dignity and rights" fails to engage with the realities of social inequity and power differentials.[17] Such rhetoric operates at a sufficient level of abstraction to provide a cover for states and other agencies that actually forestalls any real engagement with these inequities and differentials. Saudi Arabia is a signatory to CEDAW (Convention on the Elimination of All Forms of Discrimination Against Women) despite the immobility and lack of agency it imposes on its female citizens.

This abstraction in ethics and politics leaves the narrative of Man, so familiar as to be almost invisible, firmly in place. In nature humans, unlike the sociable bees, live in a state of perpetual war. Men fight over generative space—women and land—and possession depends on a man's might. The institution of sovereign power transforms might into right and possession into property. From Hobbes to Hegel, Freud, and Lévi-Strauss, in the narrative of human identity, relations among men are mediated by the laws of property and the exchange of women.

Bioethics and philosophy reflect this privileging of property and sexual propriety. "Stem cell research, genetic testing, cloning: progress in the life sciences is giving human beings new power to improve our health and control the development processes of all living species."[18] For the most part, bioethics embraces this "scientific progress" as an unalloyed good necessary to the promotion of human well-being. Contemporary bioethics focuses almost exclusively on issues that are raised by scientific research and medical practice. UNESCO's website, as well as conference programs or funding streams, indicates the privilege accorded in bioethics to issues of consent surrounding the use of new technologies in the clinic or the lab as well as concerns about the ownership of genetic material, genetic data, or the profitable results of research. Frequently, the debates in bioethics appear to be more concerned with liability and property than with ethics.[19] Moreover, these debates address issues that affect only a very small and very privileged slice of the global population.[20] Coupled with a focus on individual agency, this concern with property and "controlling the development processes of all living species" relegates to the margins a critique of the link between health and institutions of power and wealth.

In debates about the use of reproductive technologies, stem cell research, or genetic testing, bioethics' reliance on the discourse of abstract rights, as well as concepts of property and sexual propriety drawn from social contract theory, assumes a model of conflicting interests and economic competition, at the same time that it takes for granted current economic structures and distributions of power. Who has the "right" to assisted reproductive technologies?[21] Are the "rights" of the unborn violated in stem cell research or prenatal testing? Who "owns" or has a "right" to the unimplanted, fertilized embryos left over from the procedure of in vitro fertilization? Who "owns" or has a "right" to genetic data? Similarly, debates about the use of new technologies in end-of-life care are focused around rights and property. Who has a right to this care or the right to refuse or suspend this care? Who is financially liable for this care? Bioethics has often reverted to some form of cost-benefit analysis to determine whether or not the investment in end-of-life care or the treatment of rare diseases is justified. [22] Recent debates in the United States have often pitted eldercare against investments in prenatal care and child health, as if the alternative were inevitable and to be decided by an analysis of macroeconomic benefit or social cost.[23]

Bioethics tends to assume that scientific research and the development of new technologies for "controlling life" constitute positive "progress," and it focuses on resolving problems of consent or debates about rights in order to facilitate that research and technological development. Rarely does bioethics ever interrogate the aim of "controlling life" or question whether or not these scientific and technological developments actually promote human health and happiness. The complicity of bioethics with state funding and state-sanctioned committees and commissions seems to support Foucault's claim that "this is what philosophers do: He does not tell the truth about the nature of States, he tells the truth so that what is said in a State is in line with the truth of the State."[24] Bioethicists involved in the formulation of the Affordable Care Act (Obamacare), for example, supported differential restrictions not applied to other medical care on reproductive services for women as a strategic necessity to pass a bill, as if denying women access to basic health care were ethically sustainable.[25]

◆　◆　◆　◆

Against the abstract rational subject of the rights of Man and the hypothetical imperatives of moral philosophy, a critical phenomenology makes the privileging of property over life seem strange. It reveals the familiar gender division of labor to be unsustainable amidst the current claims of work and family. It gives voice to the labor of women as a starting point for philosophy and ethics. What are the ethical and political implications of the real universal that everyone is born of a woman? What are the ethical and political implications of the real universal that every human being must eat other living things, plants or animals, to survive? What ethical imperatives follow from these conditions of life?

First, an ethics and a politics that begin with women's labor make generativity the aim. Everyone is dependent on the generativity of a woman. Mothering cultivates the other's independence. Teachers, supervisors, friends, colleagues, and parents confront everyday the possibilities of generativity: the opportunity to promote the other's success and independent agency. How must the infrastructures of life be organized to enable every child to solve creatively the question of who she is, so that she can become a generative force, a mother, in her own right?

Second, an ethics of life begins not with a fiction of liberty but from the necessary interdependencies of life. Everyone is always already indebted to the ones who have come before: to the ones who took care of me when I could not take care of myself, to what I have eaten and to those who grew it and served it. The privilege of being "at liberty" depends upon an environment that I cannot secure by myself and on services that I cannot provide on my own. Thinking through these interdependencies reveals the way in which freedom depends on a *culture of possibilities.* A person who lives in a food desert in the United States is not at liberty to eat a healthy diet anymore than Saudi women are at liberty to address their obesity epidemic. Freedom depends on the creation of real opportunity and a new culture of possibilities.

Third, these interdependencies call for an ethics of collaboration focused on building solidarities in the imagination of a new future. Critical phenomenology exposes the continuities and complicities between structures of subjection in the Anglo-European sphere and in developing economies. Poor women in India are recruited as surrogate mothers because the pressure on Anglo-European women to reproduce biologically creates a robust market. Imported domestic labor from developing economies addresses the crisis in the gender division of labor as Anglo-European women move into paid work. The Saudi women who protested the ban on women driving have a claim to mobility no less than their Western sisters or any human. Uma Narayan and other scholars who criticize the gender relations of their cultures and advocate for the economic independence and political liberty of women express a universal claim that calls for transnational collaborations and solidarities.[26]

Like Saudi women, Anglo-European women are significantly underrepresented in leadership positions or decision-making bodies. They have less economic independence and social mobility than men, are more likely to be poor, and more likely to be the victims of domestic or sexual violence. Critiques of the treatment of Indian surrogates or the restrictions on Saudi women target not those cultures per se but a virtually ubiquitous narrative of property and sexual propriety that devalues women's labor and renders women invisible in public domains of action and decision. The charge that such critiques impose "Western values" denies to these women the self-consciousness that seeks agency and mobility, as if the critic were at liberty to assume, against his own autonomy and liberty, that these women must be happy in their confinement and enforced dependency. While it is important to recognize the complicity of global capital and other Anglo-European forces in the subjection of women in other cultures, it is equally important to create solidarities with those women and to be unafraid to criticize the elements of their cultures that maintain their subjection.[27]

If the infrastructures of subjection are transcultural and transnational, the critique must be also.

Finally, under an ethics of life or generativity, no one is innocent. No act can be sufficient to realize all the moral claims in play, any more than one figure of the universal will be adequate to the rich profusion of human experience. Do I spend more time caring for my patients or more time caring for my family? Do I spend more time caring for my ailing mother if it means less time with my children? Do I spend more time with the student who doesn't understand even if it means the smarter ones feel ignored? These are the quotidian quandaries of ethical life.

More extreme irreconcilabilities face women in more extreme circumstances. Do I sell my eldest daughter to a broker so that I can feed the rest of my children? The idea that reason can provide a test adequate to determine the right course of action, while preserving the self's moral purity, both misunderstands the exigencies of ethical life and perverts ethical thinking into a moral egoism. Acting according to the value of generativity and to promote life, the agent nevertheless cannot give every claim its due. Everyone will be in need of forgiveness.

The corrupting forces of ethical life are the *hardheadedness* and *hardheartedness* of sticking to one claim as if it were absolute, in denial of all the others. The hardhead who refuses to recognize that impinging moral claims cannot be resolved in an action and the hardheart who refuses to forgive the other for this lack undermine the sociality and collaboration that are essential to ethical life and to human health and happiness.

Critical phenomenology exposes the contingency of Man as a figure of the human and the possibility of imagining infrastructures of life other than property, sexual propriety, and the gender division of labor. Beginning from the real universals of our real dependencies, an ethics of life calls for the development of collaborations to build solidarities of voice and action to promote generativity, mobility, and a culture of possibilities capable of sustaining the freedom of each and all.

Acknowledgments

A BOOK THAT seeks to shift ethics and politics away from the law of property and sexual propriety toward the values of collaboration and generativity will necessarily have depended upon those values itself. Without the encouragement and advice of friends and colleagues it would never have been completed.

Wendy Lochner's enthusiasm for the project brought me across the finish line. No one ever had a better editor. Her assistant at Columbia University Press, Christine Dunbar, patiently helped me prepare the manuscript for production. I am deeply grateful to both.

Many thanks to Alyssa Adamson, Eva Boodman, Emma Velez, and Caleb Ward for their work on the footnotes and bibliography and to Kate Caras who generously volunteered to copyedit the final manuscript.

Many thanks to the London School of Hygiene and Tropical Medicine for the Fellowship in Ethics and Philosophy in 2013–14 that allowed me the time to complete the manuscript. I am indebted to John Porter, Helen Walls, Johanna Hanefeld, Ferdinand Okwaro, Sridhar Venkatapuram, Sandra Albert, and all my colleagues at LSHTM for enlightening and inspiring conversations.

Many thanks to Alexandra Villing, curator of Greek pottery and figurines, Department of Greece and Rome, British Museum, for sharing her expertise on the terra cottas of Demeter and Persephone. Given her scholarly precision and reticence, I should hasten to add that all speculations are my own.

Audiences at the University of Bergen, the University of Manchester, the University of Glasgow, Goldsmith College, University College London, University of Warwick, University of Ghent, Macquarie University, DePaul University, Miami University of Ohio, and the CUNY Graduate Center offered questions, comments, and criticisms on earlier versions of various chapters that productively informed the final text. I am particularly indebted to Elaine Miller, who, early on in the project, pressed me to clarify exactly what I meant by "life." Her challenging query has stayed with me throughout my writing.

In the midst of writing, I had the good fortune to discover an ally in Bonnie Honig. Her appreciation for my reading of Antigone renewed my confidence in the project at a critical moment. I am immensely grateful for her support.

I am indebted to my colleagues in the Irigaray Circle for their constancy and collaboration. Louise Burchill, Liz Grosz, Rebecca Hill, Sabrina Hom, Serene Khader, Ellen Mortensen, Peg Rawes, and Gail Schwab all provided criticism and encouragement when it was needed.

This book attempts an uneasy marriage of Foucault's genealogical method and Luce Irigaray's thought of the irreducibility of sexual difference. While Foucault is dead and I never knew him, Luce Irigaray is very much alive. My work would not be possible had she not blazed the trail. I hope she will see this book as a daughter's attempt to carry forward the mother's legacy.

My colleagues in FAB (International Network of Feminist Approaches to Bioethics) and *IJFAB* (*International Journal of Feminist Approaches to Bioethics*) have been a constant source of productive criticism and joyful collaboration. Françoise Baylis, Jim Dwyer, Lisa Eckenwiler, and Dafna Feinholz each offered generous support and advice when it was needed. Angus Dawson has been a willing and generous collaborator who inspired me to push the boundaries of bioethics. Wendy Rogers and Jackie Leach Scully have been the best of partners and the truest of friends. Everything I have accomplished in the last ten years has their mark on it. Regrettably, our colleague Anne Donchin is no longer here for me to thank, but the memory of her generative spirit lives on in all the women and men in bioethics that she nurtured and inspired.

My Stony Brook colleague Eva Feder Kittay not only supported *IJFAB* but also offered counsel and encouragement when it really mattered. She invited me to present an earlier version of chapter 2 in one of her seminars, and, though she may not have foreseen this, her comments were key in my development of the theme of capitalized bodies.

Late in this long run, Dick Bernstein generously volunteered to read the entire manuscript. His appreciation of the stylistic risks I took in chapter 5 gave me renewed confidence just when I was inclined to doubt.

Ellen Feder, Margrit Shildrick, and Cindy Willett read an earlier version of the manuscript, which was much improved by their incisive criticisms and constructive suggestions. All three are genuine friends who will tell me what I need to hear and who believed in the project and wanted me to succeed. I am particularly grateful to Cindy for her enthusiasm for the risks I took in basing ethics and politics on a retelling of the Demeter and Persephone myth. Her support gave me courage when I needed it.

Given that I situate food and eating at the heart of ethics, it would be remiss of me not to thank those who have fed me so well over so many years. Cyrus and Perven Todiwala of Café Spice Namasté serve the most extraordinary Indian cuisine outside India. They are passionately committed to sustainability, deeply involved in educating the public about the beauty and complexity of Indian food, and actively promote and inspire a new generation of chefs. It is an honor to call them my friends.

Jason Atherton's Pollen Street Social and Social Eating House have provided me with more exquisitely satisfying meals than I can count. In welcoming and unpretentious environments, Jason and Paul Hood serve equally unpretentious but fabulously imaginative food featuring locally sourced ingredients and an intense, creative juxtaposition of flavors and textures. While the food is brilliant, the team Jason has assembled is just as remarkable. They have been with him, as have I, from the beginning of the Social experience. Michael West, Laure Patry, Martin Renshaw, Boris Poliakov, Gareth Evans, and Kyle Wilkinson have taught me much not only about food, wine, and spirits but also about loyalty, camaraderie, and what can be accomplished together through courage and hard work. I am especially indebted to Gareth for The Professor, a signature drink that I highly recommend. Many thanks to the entire Social team for their generous and inspiring friendship.

An earlier version of chapter 3 appeared in *The Returns of Antigone*, edited by Tina Chanter and Sean D. Kirkland (SUNY Press, 2014). I am grateful to Tina and Sean for their appreciation of my reading of the oedipal plays.

An earlier version of chapter 6 appeared in *Labor and Global Justice: Essays on the Ethics of Labor Practices Under Globalization*, which I edited with Wim Vandekerckhove, Ronald M. S. Commers, and Tim R. Johnston (Lexington, 2014). I am grateful to Ronald for inspiring me to place labor at the center of ethics and politics.

Finally, last, but by no means least, I owe an infinite debt of gratitude to my husband Mark J. Sedler, M.D. and my son Alexander Crenshaw Sedler. Without their love and support, I would have accomplished nothing.

Just Life

Introduction

OUR TIME—MAN, MONEY, AND MEDIA

We are rounding off reality with a demolition project that is assuming insane proportions. . . . We can no longer set anything "against" this technological world. . . . And those who still have a glimmer of nostalgia in them are asking why the world is so vulnerable to such a project of "globalization" and why the human being is so vulnerable to this project of systematically eliminating the human. . . . There remains, also . . . the heightened expectation of the single event that would, at a stroke, unmask the enormous conspiracy in which we are immersed. . . . The Apocalypse is present, in homoeopathic doses, in each of us.

—JEAN BAUDRILLARD, *CARNIVAL AND CANNIBAL* (2010)

Our only chance today lies in a cultural and political ethics based upon sexual difference. . . . With the objective purpose of accumulating material possessions and with the subjective goal of bolstering the male subjective economy, science allows disorder and pollution to increase and funds various kinds of curative medicine. Science contributes to destruction, then repairs things as best it may. But a body that has suffered is never the same. It retains the traces of physical and moral trauma, it remembers despair, it thirsts for revenge. This whole economy is testimony to the way men have forgotten life. Vast resources are squandered for money. But what is money if it does not serve life? Despite the various pro-birth policies that nations adopt for economic or sometimes religious reasons, it is clear that destroying life is as much an imperative as giving birth.

—LUCE IRIGARAY, "A CHANCE FOR LIFE" (1986)

Money should be spent trying out concepts that shatter our current structures and systems that have turned much of the world into one vast market. Is progress really Wi-Fi on every corner? No. It's when no 13-year-old girl on the planet gets sold for sex. But as long as most folks pat themselves on the back for charitable acts, we've got a perpetual poverty machine.

—PETER BUFFETT, "THE CHARITABLE-INDUSTRIAL COMPLEX" (2013)

PHILOSOPHERS FREQUENTLY STRIKE an apocalyptic tone. Since Plato, analogies have often been made between philosophy and medicine as if philosophy, like medicine, were the response to a *krisis,* a moment of judgment determining whether the patient will live or die. Diagnosing the urgencies and ills of their times, philosophers offer their work as a necessary treatment for the body politic. By teaching others to see and think differently, philosophers not only call into question identities and principles but also reimagine them as infrastructures of life. Very few philosophers have been content merely to proclaim disaster without offering, at the same time, an ameliorating path.

No one has gone farther in diagnosing the catastrophe of our time than Jean Baudrillard. In texts written and presented in 2005, shortly before his illness and death, Baudrillard analyzes the contemporary "mutation" in human life under the shift from domination, defined by the dynamic relation between master and slave, to hegemony, the lateral circulation of an indifferent power that reduces all value in a universal market of generalized exchange. Our time is the "twilight of critical thought and the agony of power."[1] Both capital and history, Baudrillard insists, have, by a totalizing gesture, eliminated the very undecidability and irreducibility that made the rhetoric and material strategies of freedom, representation, and liberation possible. This lateralization and generalization of exchange eliminates the distinctions of markets and scales of value. Under hegemony,

the system works exponentially:
—not starting from value, but from the liquidation of value.
—nor through representation, but through the liquidation of representation.
—not from reality but from the liquidation of reality.

(49)

Whereas domination gave rise to history as the story of the slave reclaiming his freedom, hegemony exercises an internal "deterrence" that discredits in advance any historical reference and transforms reality into "parody, mockery, or masquerade" (50). Reality is swamped by infinite flows of information and media to the point that it becomes merely virtual. Rational markets governed by a law of exchange are flooded by flows of global capital, and speculation produces a "depreciation of all value" (43). At the same time, forms of democratic representation cease to function: they are inundated by "various forms of manipulation and parallel networks," as well as vast sums of money and the intimate complicities of corporate wealth and traditional democratic institutions (49).[2] The homogeneous tide of global capital sweeps aside differences of value and identity and overwhelms information and representation, at the same time that it produces dams of privilege and concentrates wealth.

This "catastrophe" involves not only political representation but also the very ability of an individual human to achieve some interiority or self-representation. "After the sacrifice of value, after the sacrifice of representation, after the sacrifice of reality, the West is now characterized by the deliberate sacrifice of everything through which a human being keeps some value in his or her own eyes" (67). Not only are all values subject to the same parodic and mimetic forces, but also the drama of desire and fulfillment in which the Western self is born has collapsed into the instantaneous. Communication, information, and commerce occur at top speed, optimally with no delay at all. Culture can be instantly downloaded. Experiences are immediately reified and distributed on digital media. Digital speed effaces the gap between desire and fulfillment, the space of identity, agency, and narrative.

This liquidation of reality and identity facilitates and maintains a moral callus sufficient to protect privilege against the spectacle of the others' suffering. Whole populations are disposed of, without outrage, as the collateral damage of the war industry or the capitalized bodies of sex trafficking or the invisible, delegitimized, and abused bodies of farmworkers or the shrink-wrapped and sanitized meat that leaves no trace of the other animals who are victims of industrialized meat production. Under the liquidation of value, nothing commands respect or resists commercialization and deregulation. Nothing looks back.

Every culture is vulnerable to appropriation by global capital. Hegemony operates through the "simulation" of all values and cultures, and this "derealization," not the "violation of rights," constitutes the failure of democratic representation (63). Las Vegas comprises Paris, the South Pacific, pharaonic Egypt, Ceasar's Rome, and King Arthur's court, all within easy walking distance of one another. Paris, on the other hand, the disposable city, disposes itself all over the world in its talismans and imitations, a *tour Eiffel* on every key chain and a bistro in every borough.[3] Places either become a brand like Paris or are branded by the global brands, Coke signs and McDonald's arches describing the horizon from one end of the world to the other.

Baudrillard links this crisis of value, representation, identity, and reality to "the West's" dominance of "the Other" through the imposition of supposedly universal values that are, in fact, specifically its own: "In the name of universals, the West imposes its political and economic models on the entire world along with its principle of technical rationality" (66).[4] Western universalism exports its politics and economics under a cancerous illusion of "unlimited growth and prosperity" that masks the real austerity of life under global capital.

At the same time, this universalism envelops the Other and others in the myth of "whiteness."[5] The undifferentiated, totalized universal of Man imposes whiteness as the zero degree of experience. Every other figure becomes a special case, an exception, a variation, or a degradation. Whiteness, without color or distinction, nonetheless absorbs all difference without differentiation.

The "white terror" of hegemony under global capital installs as universal what was originally a "cultural singularity" of the Western narrative of mastery and slavery: discrimination.[6] "The Universal is not for everyone. Only discrimination is universal."[7] The fiction of the generic subject Man, the fiction of an indifferent universal, applied everywhere, authorizes and installs systems of discrimination and criteria of qualification. It produces not only the exclusionary spaces of refugee camps and immigration detention facilities but also the heterogeneous spaces of the Persian Gulf's luxury condominiums or Western "gentrification" in which "the deepest misery and enclaves of luxury coexist in the same geographic space" (52–53). Like desire, imagination, the individual, reality, history, and rational value, the universal has passed into "obsolescence." The horizon of this "new era" of hegemony is the "obsolescence of humanity and its values" (86–87).

Against this dark closure of history, Baudrillard speculates very limited futures. An "immense work of mourning" replaces the energetic narrative of the slave's becoming free (62). Baudrillard seems to dismiss "real solidarity between nations" as an impossibility that spawns the false universal of a coalition against the "specter of Absolute Evil" (97). In place of the genuine solidarity and collaboration that Franklin D. Roosevelt makes essential to any democratic republic, nations in our time shift alliances to maximize security and protect wealth so that only the threat of Absolute Evil guarantees their bonds.[8]

Baudrillard insists, however, that as the hegemonic operation intensifies so do the points of resistances, "singularities . . . that exclude themselves from the universal and play their own game, at their own risk and peril" (102). He advances as examples of these "unexchangeable singularities" "rogue states" like Iran or Palestine, but these states seem to be caught up in the very logic of "white terror" and its systems of colonization and exclusion that Baudrillard has diagnosed (70–71). Their "counterterrorism" reinforces their exclusion from the universal, however self-willed and preemptory that exclusion may have been, and therefore from the "unlimited growth and progress" of the West. It reinscribes their identity as the Other to Man. They do not seem to be countersingularities to the logic of hegemony and the securitization of life, but powerful forces maintaining the destruction of life and the conditions of life to serve security and wealth. They do not seem to offer any escape from the liquidation of reality, identity, and value, but seem to intensify these losses. "To find the only adversary who will face this all-powerful hegemony, we must look for those beings that are strangers to will, exiled from dialogue and representation, exiled from knowledge and history" (104). Baudrillard quickly reverts to the politically oppressed—the Palestinians, for example, or the colonized peoples of Paris' *banlieu*—but this gesture only returns everything to the very logic of fraternal struggle, property, tribalism, and terror that feeds hegemony. The logic of revenge that fuels terrorism or counterterrorism belongs to Man's conflict over generative space and is no stranger to its knowledge and history.

In considering the possibility of a livable future, Baudrillard insists that "power itself must be abolished—and not solely in the refusal to be dominated, which is at the heart of all traditional [revolutionary] struggles—but also, just as violently, in the refusal to dominate (if the refusal to dominate had the same violence and the same energy as the refusal to be dominated, the dream of revolution would have disappeared long ago)" (47). Yet the relationship that has as its aim letting the other go free never crosses Baudrillard's mind.

With the philosopher's usual blindness to sexual difference, Baudrillard does not notice that even within the West, even within "whiteness," human experience has never been One. There has never been one Universal of human experience. The myth of the generic subject Man was always a deft and strategic illusion, the *presto chango* of domination through which the gender division of labor is installed. There was always, and from the very beginning, an exclusion, the trace of the two. The indifferent, totalized universal Man may be "dragged away in its distintegration" (76). It may be "vain to want to restore [Man's] universal values from the debris of globalization" (76). But, Man is not the whole of life, not even of the human.

Exiled from dialogue and representation. Known, but not the knower, in politics, science, and philosophy. The silent voice of the great narrative of the slave's becoming free. Lacking agency or even history. Perhaps women's experience and the concept of woman in the history of philosophy provide exactly the counterforces that Baudrillard and our time require.[9]

◆ ◆ ◆ ◆

In our time "the truth don't matter like it ought to."[10] In the plethora of media, the truth becomes hard to find and identify. Public debate devolves into mere factionalism. If one party supports an initiative, the other must be against it. Journalists present opposing sides as if all positions have equal value. Advertising and other self-interested discourses substitute strategies of persuasion for real argument so that sophistry drowns out truth.

In our time money serves as a generic value, as if all goods could be arrayed on the same scale. So thoroughly economized is our experience that all conversations focus on cost. Debates about health care, for example, focus not on what is needed to support human agency and community, but on payment schemes and cost containment. Wealth brings privilege, and the worth of a human life seems to be determined by its income. Work loses its intrinsic value: the point is not to be the best carpenter or physician, but to make money.

In our time, women still do not enjoy full participation in the councils that determine the future. Their labor remains undervalued and often invisible. They are often the victims of sexual or domestic violence. In many areas of the world, women still have the status of a man's property.

In our time the hegemony of media, money, and Man threatens our survival. War, environmental degradation, and the commercialization of all aspects of life threaten human health and happiness while putting all life at risk. The built environment serves capital and the war machine rather than human experience. At the same time, the factionalism and sophistry of public discourse make it almost impossible to act collectively to address the urgencies produced by the sacrifice of human welfare to economic interest.

Perhaps universals are mortal too. Perhaps Man has had his day. Perhaps it is time to begin again elsewhere, in what remains other and unspoken. Perhaps it is time, in our time, to transform how we see and think through new narratives. Perhaps our mythologies and histories offer unheard voices and invisible images. Perhaps women's experience and all that has been associated with it—nature, animality, immediacy, vulnerability, generativity, and maternal life—all that which philosophy has for millennia relegated to the margins, while mining it as a reservoir of metaphors, foils, and tropes, perhaps this shelters unheard-of universals for our time.

Perhaps new figures of (female) agency—a girl with a book, a frieze of blooming young girls, a loving sister, the intergenerational generativity of mother and daughter—may provide the "concepts that shatter our current structures and systems." Perhaps these figures may sustain modes of life beyond property, sexual propriety, and the gender division of labor.

PART ONE
Critique of Rights

Hitherto I have set forth the nature of Man, (whose Pride and other Passions have compelled him to submit himself to Government;) together with the great power of his Governor, whom I compared to *Leviathan*, taking that comparison out of the two last verses of the one and fortieth of *Job*; where God having set forth the great power of *Leviathan*, calleth him King of the Proud. *There is nothing*, saith he, *on earth, to be compared with him. He is made so as not to be afraid. Hee seeth every high thing below him; and is King of all the children of pride.*

—THOMAS HOBBES, *LEVIATHAN*, CHAPTER 28 (1651)

Western man chooses to measure himself against the terrible rather than the calm. . . . He likes to tame the infuriated sea, the wild animals, the unbridled passions. . . . Nature becomes wild, the adversary against whom he must fight. All that exists is reduced to what man must overcome. Beginning from his entry, he recreates it in order to dominate it. From this intention results the universe as violence.

—LUCE IRIGARAY, *TO BE TWO* (1994)

EVERYTHING HUMAN IN nature begins with the myth of perpetual war. While bees and ants "live sociably with one another, (which are therefore by *Aristotle* numbered amongst Political creatures;) . . . Man-kind cannot do the same."[1] Bees and ants "naturally" agree among themselves to form collaborations and alliances. The sociable bees and ants act as a swarm, a single body of many individual members that is neither incoherent in its buzzing activity nor shapeless in the shifting outlines of its constantly reassembling army. Each member of the hive or hill finds its private want in the common good of all.

Unlike these naturally civil bees and ants, men are naturally disposed to compare themselves to one another and "are continually in competition for Honor and Dignity." The members of the class "Man-kind" are bellicose *by nature* and inevitably become enemies. Each man naturally believes that he is better than the rest, wiser and more deserving. Each man assumes that he should rule the others. Their competition over land, goods, women, and power leads necessarily to "Envy and Hatred, and finally Warre." In nature men dissociate, and life is "poore, nasty, brutish, and short."[2] In nature each one violently defends his satisfying resources and violently asserts his signs of honor and power against the others. When all men do the same, an indefinite war of each against all ensues. Hobbes' myth recreates Man's natural life as a theater of perpetual violence.

Unlike the naturally civil ants and bees who swarm with one agency, men require the "terror of some power" to subdue their competing wills and impose peace. Only an awesome force could impose upon them the cooperation that is essential to their welfare, no less than to the ants and bees. To limn the scale of this power, Hobbes reaches for the Book of Job and its monstrous sea beast or dragon.[3] "Upon earth there is not his like, a creature without fear." His vast wake bathes the ocean with frost. "He makes the deep boil like a pot . . . the sea like a pot of ointment." Largest of all the animals ever to have lived on earth, the great blue whale (*balaenoptera musculus*) reaches 80 to 100 feet in length and weighs between 110 and 190 tons, similar in size and shape to the fuselage of a Boeing 737. Naturally graceful swimmers, cleaving and breaching the sea with a gentle elegance, few animals display such speed and power as Leviathan when threatened. English whaling flourished in the first half of the seventeenth century, and Hobbes must have been familiar with tales of its harrowing dangers. Boats might be crushed or plunged to the depths of the ocean or dragged so far out to sea that the whalers could not find the way back to their ship. Both the immense value of a whale as a commodity and its awesome power in a fight fit the scale of sovereign power. It has no fear of Man, but men will learn to be afraid of it.

Exactly two centuries after Hobbes, another author conjures the terrible might of this colossal animal to test the limits of sovereign power. Maritime life has always been governed by a principle of absolute and inviolable sovereignty. Mutiny is a crime, however bad the captain. Like the hive and the hill, the ship depends on its members acting with one purpose. The captain, literally the head of this aggregate body, moves others by his words or commands to work toward the ship's aim. "They were one man, not thirty . . . all varieties were welded into oneness, and were all directed to that fatal goal which Ahab their one lord and keel did point to."[4]

Sovereign power may transform conflict into collaboration: it may make the aggregate body of the crew "one man." As power, however, it has its own pride. Sovereign power is no more exempt from "Envy and Hatred" than any other power. Sovereigns fall into conflict and their subjects suffer. Ahab, consumed by hate and pride, by the need to prove his own sovereignty, ignores the duties of the ship, risking it and his crew in his relentless battle. Ahab goads the whale until it turns his ship into a hearse. Is a bad sovereign better than none at all? When does the sovereign's failure to protect his subjects absolve them of their obedience?[5]

If it is natural for men to be enemies and to fight over goods, women, and recognition, it is nonetheless also "natural" and "rational" for them to make peace by submitting to the authority of some governing power mighty enough to control them all. Men submit to sovereign power only because it is in their self-interest to be delivered from the reliance on their own might and the constant threat of violence. Hobbes' story of the origin of civil society focuses on this necessity of transforming possession by might into possession by right. Under sovereign power, disputes among men do not cease to arise: men continue to be subject to competition, envy, and hatred. Man's selfish, prideful nature persists in civil society, but his conflicts with other men are resolved not by random violence and war but by the adjudication of the sovereign power. In Hobbes' narrative of political life, Man emerges when each man exchanges his *natural* rights for the "artificial" *civil* rights guaranteed to each and all by the ruling sovereign. Man's motivating passion for this exchange, and thus the mainspring of civil society, is the "Feare of Death."[6] Man exchanges the ubiquitous fear of death in the perpetual war of nature for the regularized fear of death under the law of sovereign power.

A century and a half later, political philosophy still adheres to Hobbes' storyline. When it comes to Man, natural life offers perpetual war, a scene of violence and domination. Rather than distinguishing Man from the naturally civil bees and ants, Hegel invokes, as his paradigm of natural life, the natural antagonism of the eagle and the rabbit. Nature divides itself into predators and prey. The identity of animals is determined by their *differentiae*: tooth and claw for the hunter, the means of escape for the hunted.[7] The eagle's very body—eye, beak, and talon—prescribes its destiny to eat the rabbit, as the rabbit's strong haunches and speed to ground signify its destiny as prey. The eagle rules because he can and must. Within this domain there is no right, only might.

In the myth of prehistory that opens the analysis of self-consciousness in the *Phenomenology of Spirit*, solitary men in nature enjoy an absolute sovereignty over its goods and themselves. When a man encounters another man, however, a fight ensues in which "each seeks the death of the other," while each one undertakes the "staking of its own life."[8] In this mythology, history again begins with subjection: mastery and slavery provide the initial figuration of civil life. In the violent encounter someone risks his life absolutely, while the other gives in and submits himself and his assets to his conqueror as the conqueror's property. Hegel's narrative adheres to Hobbes': right, civil society, and the state originate in this moment of servitude to the fear of death.

Within these founding stories of social and political life, women appear only as the property of men. Excepting a discussion of the marriage of priests, in which he argues against the position that the "use of Wives" is contrary to chastity, Hobbes hardly acknowledges that a female sex exists.[9] Clearly, nature is marked feminine against the masculine authority of the state.[10] In discussing the family, however, Hobbes makes no mention of women at all. A family constitutes a "little Monarchy; whether that Family consist of a man and his children; or of a man and his servants; or of a man, and his children, and servants together: wherein the Father or Master is the Sovereign."[11] It is as if this sovereign were capable of reproducing on his own, without need of a woman. Rendering women invisible, Hobbes appropriates her generativity for the male subject, just as he appropriates the generativity of nature itself for the Sovereign. Woman will be the paradigm of property and the medium of fraternal exchange.

Hegel, on the other hand, discourses at length on women. Indeed, he makes the difference between man and woman the originary figure of social and political life.[12] Women will play an essential role in sustaining the state by staying at home to tend the body and the blood: bearing and caring for children, feeding the family, tending the sick and the elderly, and burying the dead. Her activity frees a man from bodily need, so that he can be free to pursue the discursive activities of science, politics, and philosophy. In Hegel's myth of origin, sexual difference is, first and foremost, a division of labor. And women's labor necessarily belongs to men. She remains his property and the medium of his regeneration and fraternal exchange. Moreover, though she is spoken about, she cannot speak for herself and remains invisible in the spheres of political life.

These themes then—the discontinuity of natural and civil life, the inherently violent nature of Man, the necessity of some form of sovereignty or mastery to keep that nature in check, the transformation of might into right, the status of women as property, and the invisibility of women in the public arenas where decisions about the community's future are made—form a tight narrative web that still binds us today. The discourse of rights still reflects its origin in the right to property and norms of sexual propriety.[13]

Today the commodification of existence seems almost complete: social hierarchies are determined by wealth, and everything, even life itself, has a price tag. At the same time, debates rage around sexual identity and women's generativity. In some countries women are murdered for daring to love outside their tribe, while in the United States women are deprived of reproductive services or find themselves subjected to interrogations or invasive procedures when attempting to exercise their constitutional right to terminate an unwanted pregnancy. Men who fail to fulfill the role of the "little Monarch," who dare to love other men or wish to live as women, are abused or murdered in the name of sexual propriety.

Man has had his day.[14] Concepts are no more immortal than a man himself. As Derrida remarked in another context, concepts "work themselves to a point of exhaustion."[15] No doubt, at certain times and places, the rallying cry of the rights of Man has proved a shield for the vulnerable. More often, however, the invocation of rights has been tied to privilege. In his 1817 Inaugural Address celebrating the liberty of the American citizen, James Monroe posed the rhetorical question: "On whom has oppression fallen in any quarter of our Union? Who has been deprived of any right?" He did not expect an answer, nor did his audience give him one. Under a government that "protected every citizen in the full enjoyment of his rights," women, slaves, and men who held no property were invisible and excluded from the arenas of speech where decisions about the future were made.[16]

Today, this invisibility continues: women of all races, the poor, and men of color are dramatically underrepresented in the bodies that make decisions about their futures. Rather than protecting the vulnerable and promoting their agency, the discourse of rights, in its abstraction and focus on property, more likely supplies a cover for injustice and social inequity. Perhaps disentangling the web of this narrative will expose both its complicity in social and sexual inequity and the positive possibility of starting elsewhere. Justice requires an interrogation of the "we" of philosophy and its exclusions. Justice requires a critique of abstract names as powers of classification and disposition. Justice requires an analysis of the authority to command. Justice requires an intervention at the incandescent surface where the power of the name or command meets the flesh of a living human body. Justice requires not only a redistribution of goods but "changing the laws of language" with other names and declarations than Man's.[17]

Perhaps, after this interrogation of Man, it will be time to begin again, in what remains other and unspoken in the narrative of rights. The concepts, principles, and forms generated from women's experience, from a different relation to others and to nature, will be no less universal than Man's. The philosophical project of universalizing these experiences will require new stories of origin, new names and figures of agency, new institutions and forms of authority and respect. Perhaps, after the interrogation, it will be possible to imagine a collaboration that does not depend on property, power, and the fear of death.

The whale resurfaces. Ahab gives the command.

I

State of Nature!

PROPERTY, PROPRIETY, AND THE RIGHTS OF MAN

The true founder of civil society was the first man who, having enclosed a piece of land, thought of saying, "this is mine."
—JEAN-JACQUES ROUSSEAU, *DISCOURSE ON INEQUALITY*, PART 2 (1755)

Woman is the Eternal Irony of the Community.
—G. W. F. HEGEL, *PHENOMENOLOGY OF SPIRIT* (1807)

A CENTURY AFTER Hobbes, the narrative of Man's transition from the state of nature to civil life via a contract or covenant is available to Rousseau as an artifact ready to hand and widely distributed. Man's unique differences from other living creatures give rise to both the necessity and the possibility of the covenant. All living creatures, stimulated by sense, act on appetite to achieve satisfaction and avoid pain. Man, however, unlike other animals, finds his natural state intolerable. More avaricious than other animals, he does not, like the bee, naturally identify his self-interest with the social formation of a communal hive where goods are shared in common or distributed for the good of the whole. Each man conflicts with other men over women, land, and other objects of desire, making the state of nature a scene of perpetual violence. Man lives in perpetual fear that he will be dispossessed or killed.

This is the moment of necessity.

This fear for his goods and person motivates a man to enter into a contract with other men to secure by *right* what in nature he can possess only by *might*.

The covenant can secure peace among men only by installing the "terror of some power" to protect property, assign rights, and adjudicate conflict. Man is able to transgress nature in this way, entering into a nonnatural, "artificial" relation with the "Artificial Person" of the sovereign power only because he is distinguished from other animals by the use of speech. Bees communicate effectively without speech, and, though men do use speech as a means of communication, it is not this ability that makes humans exceptional among other living creatures. Specifically, speech invests Man with a unique power of abstraction by which he detaches from the immediacy of natural appetite and natural life so as to reduce the plurality of particulars in nature to classes and kinds and the specificity of events to general laws. Speech allows Man to think beyond appetite and immediate interest to the prudent future of the contract that promises safety and satisfaction in exchange for obedience. Abstracting from his natural right to protect his person and to satisfy his desires in any way he can, assenting to the contract, he becomes a citizen under the law like any other, an abstract person protected in his civil rights by sovereign power.

This is the moment of possibility.

But when was this assent given? Who was party to the contract? Who was allowed to speak, and who was spoken for?

THE ENDEAVOR: HOBBES ON LIFE
AND MAN'S NATURE

There is no such thing as perpetuall Tranquility of mind, while we live here; because Life it selfe is but Motion, and can never be without Desire, nor without Feare, nor more than without Sense.
—THOMAS HOBBES, *LEVIATHAN*, CHAPTER 6 (1651)

The comparison of the life of man to a race . . . holdeth so well. . . . But this race we must suppose to have no other goal, nor other garland, but being foremost . . . to endeavor is appetite . . . to be weary despair. Continually to be out-gone is misery. Continually to out-go the next before is felicity. And to forsake the course is to die."
—THOMAS HOBBES, *THE ELEMENTS OF LAW*, CHAPTER 9 (1640)

All animal life, Hobbes argues, exhibits two kinds of motion. "Vital motion," such as breathing or the circulation of the blood, is automatic and requires no "help of Imagination." "Animal or Voluntary motion," however, such as running, striking out, or otherwise moving the parts of the body, depends on "precedent thought," an active imagining of what actions are possible and what their results might be.[1] This "Endeavour," the internal action of imagination that precedes visible action, is put in motion by "Appetite or Desire." Thought belongs to "what you would have" to the desired object "which we ayme at."[2] Man is animated by the desire for or fear of objects, and thought, like life itself, consists in the endeavor to maximize the satisfaction of appetite and minimize threat.

Men, like other animals, are creatures of sense and passion, animated by basic appetites of hunger, thirst, lust, and anger. Encountering an object of sense stimulates in a man a "conception" in which the object is experienced as attractive or repulsive. The encounter produces an appetite or aversion, and this in turn produces "deliberation." As appetites and aversions continually arise in the living body, men imagine alternative courses of action in the hope of satisfaction and from the fear of deprivation. "The whole summe of Desires, Aversions, Hopes, and Fears, continued till the thing be either done, or thought impossible, is that we call *Deliberation*."[3] Deliberation terminates in action and is called *deliberation* because it "puts an end to the *Liberty* we had of doing, or omitting, according to our own Appetite, or Aversion."[4] Will is simply the final appetite or aversion adhering to the action, not a separate faculty, but embodied in and determined by the action itself.

As the very form of experience, deliberation reveals the imbrication of the past and future in the immediacy of the perceptual present. To the first conception of *sense*, memory adds a second conception of *value* in which the first is compared to other experiences and evaluated with respect to pleasure and pain as desirable or aversive. That which a man desires he wants to possess; that which he fears he wishes to eliminate. In addition to the first conception of sense and the second conception of value, a man produces a third kind of conception, an *expectation* of the consequences of imagined actions, an image of the future. Appetite and fear are anticipations of the future.[5] Every experience involves this complex temporality in which the present sense is informed by memory to produce an attitude toward the future, an expectation and intention. Perception, the immediate apprehension of an object of sense, invokes a memorial survey of similar past experiences that produces an image of a future action through which the object will be possessed or annihilated. What has been and what will be always already determine the immediacy of the perceptual now.

In deliberation, Hobbes argues, the will is not voluntary, because it is determined by these conceptions of perception, memory, and expectation and by the complex temporality that they install. The "will to do is appetite," and the "will to omit, fear."[6] Appetites and fears are caused by the conceptions or expectations of "reward and punishment," which are based on the accrued memory of the consequences of action in similar circumstances. Appetite and fear, in turn, produce motion or "voluntary action." These dispositions of the mind move the body of a man, so that he may act on other bodies, using them to satisfy his appetites or eliminating them to remove a threat.

Thinking, this activity of imagining consequences in relation to the endeavor of satisfying appetite or desire is not distinctive to man, for "Beasts also Deliberate . . . [and] must necessarily also have will."[7] Desiring some outcome, whether the attainment of a satisfying good or the avoidance of a painful harm, other animals are capable of considering and deciding among alternative courses of action by which the desired result might be produced, just as men do. Other animals also share with men memory and the capacity to learn from experience. Like men, they can approach a present situation in the light of some similar past event so as to make inferences about possible outcomes. Forethought or prudence combines memory with imagination to determine action, and "it is not Prudence that distinguisheth man from beast" (chapter 3, 23). Neither for Man nor beast is there any autonomy of the imagination from the demands of appetite nor any thought of the future except the prudent decision on how to satisfy it. Correlatively, other entities are neither good nor evil in themselves, but only determined in their worth in relation to appetite and aversion. What satisfies Man's desires is good; what impedes that satisfaction or threatens him and produces fear is evil (chapter 6, 39). Nature provides a scene for the enactment of Man's desires and fears.

Man's essentially appetitive nature produces a competition among men for "Riches, Honour, Command," and this inclines men to "Contention, Enmity, and War" (chapter 11, 70). The only way for a man to secure his interest and satisfy his desires is "to kill, subdue, supplant, or repell the other." In the state of nature, there is no "*Mine* and *Thine*"; possession of goods and power over others depends on a man's own might (chapter 13, 90). Thus he lives constantly subject to the fear of violence. As soon as a man has secured his dominion over land, women, and other men, a stronger or cleverer man may come to claim it from him. In the state of nature, man has no appeal and nothing to rely on but his own strength and cunning.

The "law of nature," which is also a law of *reason,* prescribes that "a man is forbidden to do, that, which is destructive of his life, or taketh away the means of preserving the same" (chapter 14, 91). *Natural* right authorizes a man to "use all means and do whatsoever action is necessary for the preservation of his body."[8] Thus the concept of right originates in the fear of death and in the aim of self-preservation.[9] Right emerges in a theater of action where Man's imagination serves his appetite and his fear, his desire to possess or his will to annihilate.

Man's *natural* right extends to all the goods of nature that may satisfy his desires or protect him from threat. Even "another's body" is rightfully his to command or dispose of. The violence of the state of nature derives from the irony that all men *equally* possess this absolute right to the goods of nature and to dispose of threats.[10] Neither his senses nor his capacity for deliberation distinguishes a man from other men so as to privilege his right over that of the others. Each man enjoys a right to "possess, use, and enjoy all things he will and can, and to do whatever he will to whomever he will," but the right proves useless, for there is "little use and benefit of the right a man hath, when another as strong, or stronger than himself, hath right to the same."[11] Man's natural right to desired goods and his natural liberty to do whatever he pleases to protect and satisfy himself produces in nature a "condition of Warre of every one against everyone."[12]

Hobbes likens war to "Foule weather" with which it shares a temporality of "disposition." Foul weather consists not in an actual shower of rain, but in an "inclination therto of many dayes together." The "notion of *Time*" determines war as it does the weather. War consists not only in actual battles or violence but also, even in their absence, in the disposition to fight (chapter 13, 88–89). In the state of nature, where right is might and all men have an equally absolute right to the goods of nature and to dispose of one another, violence or war is inevitable, as there exists no other power to adjudicate their inevitable conflict over the desirable objects of food, land, and women. Every man is the enemy of every other, and "the life of man, solitary, poore, nasty, brutish, and short" (89). Even in the absence of actual violence, all of man's energy and wit goes to securing his safety and basic needs, so that invention cannot be turned to industry or a culture of knowledge.

In describing this natural state of war, Hobbes admits that he is purveying myth, not history. "It may peradventure be thought, there was never such a time, nor condition of Warre as this; and I believe it was never generally so, over all the world" (89). Having cast Man as a self-interested creature thoroughly determined by his appetites and fears, Hobbes imagines what *would be* or *must have been* the case in the absence of any power other than violence for resolving the conflicts he takes to be inevitable. Man's greedy nature makes impossible strategies of sharing or collaboration. Nature, according to the myth, "dissociates" men, for it would be *contrary to reason* for man to limit his claim to desirable objects or to place a check on his instinct for self-preservation. Both generosity and solidarity are contrary to a man's interest and hence *irrational* in the state of nature.

Having inferred the myth from his analysis of man's appetitive or passionate nature, Hobbes adduces two types of evidence from experience in its support. First, he refers to common actions of his fellow Anglo-Europeans that imply an expectation of violence from other men. When taking a journey, a man tends to his security: he goes armed and well protected lest he be attacked. When a man goes to sleep, he locks his doors lest an intruder find his way in and cause harm. When at home, he keeps his chests locked lest his "children and servants" steal from him. "Does he not there as much accuse mankind by his actions," Hobbes asks, "as I do by my words?" (89). Even when civil law does exist and men know that they can rely on the law for redress and on officers of the law for protection, they still behave in ways that reflect their natural relation of distrust and conflict with other men.

The second type of evidence from experience that Hobbes repeatedly adduces in support of the myth casts non-European civilizations as "savages" permanently existing in the state of nature. The "savage people in many places of *America*" lack any form of self-government except that of the family, which depends on "natural lust" (89). "We," white European men, Hobbes insists, differ from these "savages" in the possession of culture. First and foremost, mathematics and geometry make possible the reckoning of time and the manipulation of space, so that Man can regulate the actions of men and create a built environment that answers to his appetites and fears. These sciences also enable Man to map the earth and the seas, so that he can engage in conquest and trade. Second, European life is distinguished by arts, letters, and the leisure of society, wherein men, like Hobbes—more or less freed from the fear of death and carnal appetite, as these needs are met by civil powers, servants, and wives—enjoy the opportunity to fashion narratives of the human. They trade these narratives among themselves while also imposing them on others, like the "savages" of the Americas.

The historical and cultural inaccuracy of Hobbes' claims about the diverse native peoples of the Americas can hardly be exaggerated. These peoples possessed complex calendars and clocks. Many of them built monuments to rival the Egyptian pyramids or European cathedrals. Their cultures included elaborate narratives of origin and highly articulated theologies. A subtle and detailed knowledge of nature made life sustainable and rich. Without that knowledge, the early white settlers of the Mayflower colony would have died, as their own knowledge was entirely inadequate to their need.[13] Hobbes' ill-informed assumptions about the culture of these "savages" valorized European culture against the supposed lack of it in "the wildest of the Indians." This exclusion of the "savages" from "culture" provides a strategic move in his installation of Man as the figure of the human. These are not men, not instances of Man, but "savages," and they represent the violence of liberty in nature that Hobbes' political philosophy will contain and subject.

COVENANT, "OUR BEST ENDEAVOUR": SPEECH, DEATH, AND THE MYTH OF ASSENT

The Passions that incline men to Peace, are Feare of Death; Desire of such things as are necessary to commodious living; and a Hope by their Industry to obtain them.

—THOMAS HOBBES, *LEVIATHAN*, CHAPTER 12 (1651)

Amongst masterless men, there is perpetuall war. . . .
—THOMAS HOBBES, *LEVIATHAN*, CHAPTER 21

Man is an animal who, if he lives among others of his kind, *needs a master.* . . .
One cannot fashion something absolutely straight from wood as crooked as that
of which man is made.
—IMMANUEL KANT, "IDEA FOR A UNIVERSAL HISTORY WITH
COSMOPOLITAN INTENT" (1784)

Given the unsustainably brutal and violent life of Man in the state of nature,
wherein neither a man nor his property is safe from an assault by other men,
men are motivated to seek peace. The law of nature decrees that a man will and
must do whatever is necessary to secure his person and goods. The interest of
self-preservation or the fear of death provides the motive force for the transition
from natural life to civil life. Out of rational self-interest, a man "lays down" or
divests himself of his absolute natural right and absolute natural liberty in favor
of a limited *civil* right guaranteed by a sovereign power.

In "laying down" his absolute right, a man counts on a reciprocal action from
all others. He retains for himself "only so much liberty against other men, as he
would allow other men against himself" (chapter 14, 92). The action of laying
down his absolute right can be rational, that is, not contrary to his appetite and
self-preservation, only if it is performed mutually by each and all. A man does
not "renounce" his absolute natural right and liberty: that would be irrational.
He accepts limits on his right and liberty only insofar as other men have done
the same. Moreover, some rights are inalienable and cannot be laid down. A man
seeks peace and accepts limitation on his natural right and natural liberty only
out of rational self-interest; therefore he cannot lay down the right of resisting
those who threaten his life or person.[14]

Through this "mutual transferring of right," a man enters into a "contract"
with other men to secure peace for their mutual safety and satisfaction. The
contracts that establish peace or civil life depend, not on the conceptions of
sense, but on a representation of the past and future that can take place only in
words. Some contracts are executed in the present, as when a sum of money is
exchanged for some good. The contract is completed in the present with no debt
or obligation left outstanding. The contracts that establish the mutual transfer-

ring of right, however, are not of this type, as these contracts oblige the parties to engage in future actions based on past promises. The contract enjoins a man not to some particular action but to a *course* of action. The man who enters into the social contract makes an enduring promise to forbear indefinitely from re-lapsing into the natural state of war. He promises, *as long as others do the same,* not to reclaim his absolute right to the goods of nature, nor his absolute liberty to do as he will to other men. The contract depends on Man's ability to make a promise by predicting himself: "*I will do.*" Man differentiates himself from other animals and ameliorates his brutal natural life by exploiting the power of speech to traverse time. The first origin of Man, his dissociative nature, is displaced by a second, his ability to use speech not just to communicate but to promise, pre-dict, and pronounce.

This power of speech distinguishes Man from other animals because in it he transcends the present. Speech constitutes the source of Man's dominion over other creatures and the natural world as well as the possibility of a contract to se-cure peace. It will supply the infrastructure for the system of signs wherein power is embodied and deployed. But the "first use of names," or words, is to serve as "*Markes* or *Notes* of remembrance" (chapter 4, 25). Other animals have memory sufficient for prudent action, but no way of fixing and retaining experience. As memory fades, the animal must learn again what experience has taught it.

"Whereas there is no other Felicity of Beasts, but the enjoying of their quo-tidian Food, Ease, and Lusts, as having little, or no foresight of the time to come, for want of observation, and memory of the order, consequence, and depen-dence of the things they see; Man observeth how one Event hath been produced by another; and remembreth in them Antecedent and Consequence" (chap-ter 12, 76).

By transforming experience into words, Man possesses what he has learned in the past, so that he need not labor to learn it again. From the observation of particular events and experiences, Man produces common names and "generall Rules" that enable him to imagine and manage the future. When he encounters an object similar to one in the past in its stimulation of appetite or fear, he can rely on the principles of dependence and consequence that he has learned to determine his will and guide his action. Whereas animals have only sense and memory and are capable only of knowledge of fact, "which is a thing past, and irrevocable," man is capable of "*Science . . .* the knowledge of Consequences, and dependence of one fact upon another: by which, out of that we can presently do, we know how to do something else when we will, or the like, another time" (35). Man's distinctive capacity proves to be a technique, speech, for remembering the past as way of imagining / managing the future. The naturally *involuntary* will has been transformed into a *voluntary* will when its actions no longer reflect the "last appetite or fear." Through the mastery of experience in words, a voluntary will relies on its own acquired names and principles to imagine, assess, and act on the future. Only a will that has transcended the immediacy of appetite and fear through the discipline of names and principles can be said to be voluntary. Such a will defers both appetite and action: no longer determined by the last appetite, it is regulated by a coherent image of the future produced and sustained by classifying names and a knowledge of principles. The names and principles still serve appetite and fear, mastering them only as a means of satisfying them *in the end.*[15]

To this detachment from immediacy, from the present, from appetite and fear, Hobbes adds the condition that a voluntary will may not be guided by opinion. He admits the truth of the common saying that the "world is governed by opinion."[16] He emphasizes again that even the voluntary will serves appetite and fear: it serves them more effectively than the involuntary will through its capacity to traverse time. All our actions, however futile, attempt to obtain "benefit" and avoid "harm." Words themselves become values in this attempt. Words take on the power to *cause* appetite and fear. Those who are led by opinion to believe in "the propounding of benefits and harms" envision a future in which these benefits actually do accrue. Hobbes's analysis anticipates the vast contemporary industries that exist to manipulate opinion in order to produce certain actions in the crowd. While speech distinguished Man or the human, the power of speech to control men's thoughts and actions appears to be differentially allocated among humans, and those differences produce relations of command and control. The generic Man of principle, under whose aegis "all men reason the same," is disfigured, *as a generic,* by this hierarchical differentiation between those who lack a voluntary will or are slaves to opinion and the opinionators.

At the same time that science or knowledge of consequences produces a principled approach to future satisfaction, as well as the problem of opinion, it also generates the distinctly human emotion of anxiety. Assuming that everything has a cause and every cause a result, Man exists in a "perpetuall solicitude of the time to come." To the extent that dependencies and consequences remain obscure to him, though he be sure of their existence, "that man, which looks too far before him, in the care of future time, hath his heart all the day long, gnawed on by feare of death, poverty, or other calamity; and has no repose, nor pause of his anxiety, but in sleep."[17] Too much imagination proves as dangerous as too little. A man must be able to imagine the future only so far as it increases his power to address his fears and appetites. Excess in his image of the future only brings a man back to his own (fear of) death.

Counter to this fear and the differences among men revealed by the critique of opinion, Hobbes imagines a moment of absolute reciprocity. Each man recognizes the futility of life in the state of nature, a knowledge gained from experience and fixed in speech as an acquired property. As long as men continue to rely, each one, on his own might, as long as each man continues to invoke his absolute liberty and his absolute right to the goods of nature, there will be war, and life will be "solitary, poore, nasty, brutish, and short." Man emerges to secure the species from a barren, brutal future. In the state of nature, violence is never adequate, neither to attain satisfaction nor to allay fear. Against this image, Hobbes imagines a state not without its own violence, but as a place where violence will occur *according to principle.* The anxious speaker who is "the same in all men" arises out of the difference between these two images of the future. On behalf of or in the place of natural men, Hobbes imagines an "artificial" future produced by a moment of reciprocal consent, in which each and all engage in a "mutual transferring of right." The futility of the future in the state of nature can only be ameliorated by each man's own declaration that he will forego his absolute right *if others do the same.* In this mythic moment of consent, the "wills of many concur."[18] A secure future depends on this mutual promise: it installs an indefinite commitment on the part of each and all to yield to a general will that acts on behalf of all and no one in particular.

With his gimlet eye, Hobbes envisions a future where "the terror of some power" proves necessary to secure safety and satisfaction. Men will not keep their promises unless a power exists strong enough to compel them and to "keep them in awe."[19] What was first represented as a moment of reciprocal consent among equal men now appears as a moment of synthesis that produces an entirely new being / power. In this second figuration of the transition from the state of nature to rational life or life under principles, men transfer their natural rights to an "Artificial Man," so that he may rule over all.

"Conferring all their power and strength upon one Man," they "reduce all their Wills, by plurality of voices, unto one Will." Men declare, together at once, that they, each and all, will abide by the will of the "Artificial Man," who embodies not only the power of might but also the power of speech and principle: to name, to decree, to judge. The consent of the contract yields the command of the "Covenant." Each one gives up his right to govern himself and declares, "every man with every man," to submit himself to *Sovereigne Power.*" The fear of death motivates the Covenant with Sovereign Power as the power of life and death. An "Artificial Man," however, may prove to be little different from a real man. Like Ahab, a sovereign has his own pride and envy. Like Ahab, he risks the security and wealth of his subjects in campaigns of conquest that, as Hobbes notes, are more often about honor than about security or wealth.

Peace requires not the mere absence of battle or violence, but a state in which no one is disposed to fight: first, because the punishment for violence serves as an adequate deterrent; second, because this punishment is meted out, by *right,* by a power greater than his own and that of other men. Ruling by the right of the Covenant, the declared promise of "every man with every man," sovereign power exercises the *right* to adjudicate and to assign *right,* and it enforces its authority through *legitimate* or *legalized* violence. Through "terror," sovereign power achieves conformity of "the wills of them all." Peace or this conformity of wills depends on "mutual fear." Unlike the barren anxiety of the state of nature, the shared fear of sovereign power gives birth to the "body politic,"[20] of which individual men are only particles.

In Hobbes' famous frontispiece to *Leviathan*, the solitary man at liberty in the state of nature has been absorbed into the organized swarm of the sovereign's body. Each member of the mass turns his face toward the face of the sovereign in a sign of his subjection to sovereign power. Now, like the bees, men swarm in collective action and identify their interests with the "common good" in virtue of their terror of the "Artificial Person" to which they have themselves given birth. As his body, the swarm or mass carries out the sovereign's intentions and commands as if they were his own limbs. As the head or captain of the swarm of the body politic, sovereign power holds the power of life and death in his right hand and the power of exclusion or excommunication in his left. With these two forces, the sovereign keeps the swarm in line and, moving them to work by his command, stands over the landscape of country and town like a giant,[21] rivaling the magnitude of the great *Leviathan.*

The sovereign power will determine what is *proper* to a man, "what goods he may enjoy, and what Actions he may doe, without being molested by any of his fellow Subjects."[22] Rights discourse invokes respect, not for "the whole person, but rather certain aspects of their lives—the freedom to own property . . . and make contracts, for example."[23] Onto the differences in "Wit" that make some men the slave of opinion and others the masters of persuasion, that make some capable of science and others more like the prudent beasts, Hobbes grafts differences in *Propriety,* differences both in property and in what is proper to a man in the system of signs where power is deployed. Sovereign power authorizes these differences in property and power and maintains them through the awesome and terrible violence it can apply.

The mythology of consent extends even to those who submit under conquest. Among the "Vanquished," Hobbes distinguishes between prisoners of war, who retain their liberty and with it the right to "break their bonds" and even to "kill, or carry away captive their Master," and those who, in order to "avoid the present stroke of death," declare their submission to the victor. This declaration reconstitutes a man as "Servant" whose "body" and "life" are no longer his own, whose "body" and "life" are at the disposal of the "Master" for his "use" and "pleasure." It is not the conquest that makes a man a servant, "but his own Covenant."[24] The fact that he entered into the promise only out of the fear of death provides no counterargument, Hobbes insists, as the covenant that establishes sovereign power in the first place always rests on the fear of death. Servitude transforms a man into a possession, dispossessing him of his agency and property, which belong to the master. Hobbes emphasizes the propriety of the master's declaration that the slave is *his:* both the slave's body and his property are at the disposal of the master. He may dispose of the servant, even selling him or giving him away, as he might any other property. Even military conquest does not undermine the fiction of consent.

The covenant that substitutes right for liberty and law for might depends on a mythic past that never was and an indefinite future that can never be fully determined. Without words to represent what is not present and can never be, to provide the medium of exchange in which men declare themselves and record their promises to other men, there would be "neither Common-wealth, nor Society, nor Contract, nor Peace, no more than amongst Lyons, Bears, and Wolves."[25] The declaration in speech of the indefinite promise limits men's liberty and puts an end to the violence of nature, substituting for it the awesome violence of the sovereign power's right and law. "All men reason alike," abandoning absolute liberty in favor of a more secure future of safety and satisfaction under sovereign power.

Perhaps, the declaration was coerced or never made. Perhaps, this exchange of liberty for security never was reciprocal. And, if all men reasoned alike, there would not be those differences of "Wit," which make some the masters of opinion and others mastered by it, some wealthy in property and power, others the servants of that wealth. This subjection and servitude disfigured the image of reciprocity from the very beginning, from the moment of consent itself. There never was a moment in which each and all enjoyed an equal liberty to consent. Life may be a race, but the runners do not start at the same line, nor carry the same burdens.

Beyond the inequity among men, which is part of the architecture of rights from the very beginning, lie all those who cannot fit the image of Man and do not belong to the class of "all men who reason alike." The "We" of the community of Man excludes those creatures who lack the capacity for principled thought: children, madmen, women, savages. To be named "woman" or "savage" is to be excluded from the practices and decisions in which the community's future is determined. Lacking Man's reason, women and savages could never be party to the covenant and its rights.[26]

THE POWER TO NAME: ABSTRACTION IN THE DISCOURSE OF RIGHTS

Man seems to have wanted, directly or indirectly, to give the universe his own gender, as he has wanted to give his own name to his children, his wife, his possessions.
—LUCE IRIGARAY, *JE, TU, NOUS* (1990)

All men by nature reason alike.
—THOMAS HOBBES, *LEVIATHAN*, CHAPTER 5

The most important feature of speech, that which constitutes the absolute difference of man from other animals, is its power of abstraction. Through the use of common names, man can subsume a diversity of particular things under a single identity, so that actual beings are transformed into instances of a kind. Similarly, though men and "beasts" share the ability to assess a situation in the light of experience, consider alternatives, and elect a course of action most likely to satisfy an appetite or avoid a harm, men have the capacity to abstract from the particular situation and "seek all the possible effects, that can be produced [by an action]."[27] Through words, a man acquires the ability to think beyond the particular experience to other possible scenes of action not immediately impinging upon him. Finally, through the combination of general names, Man can abstract from experience to produce "generall Rules" that both explain and predict particular cases.[28]

This power of abstraction gives rise to a "*Seeking*" or "hunting" after cause and effect that "exceedeth the short vehemence of any carnall Pleasure."[29] While animals deliberate only in relation to the satisfaction of immediate appetites, Man's "Lust of the mind" propels him to enquire into the causes and laws of all things and phenomena. Speech enables Man to abstract from the particulars of experience, subsuming them in concepts and laws. Speech also provides Man with the power to abstract from his own experience in order to represent himself as transcending the logic of sensual appetite and desire. Just as the concepts of the botanical table reduce actual living plants in nature to mere instances of a kind, so too, through the articulation of the concept of Man and its related concepts—savages, nature, woman—men are reduced to instances of the general figures of the citizen or man of reason.

The subject of rights is an abstract universal person, but this abstraction is produced through a complex of exclusions.[30] Whatever historical moment might be identified as the moment of assent, not all those governed by the contract were parties to it—not even all the men, not even all the white men. The mythology of consent invokes a moment when a promise is made among *all those who will be subject to it*, but women, savages, and children never enjoyed any absolute liberty to yield in the first place. The myth of the covenant secures Man's claim to the generic, installing Man as the figure of the human through a power of exclusion carried out by abstract names. Through abstract names and their power of disposition, actual men and women are rendered disposable, identified as nodes for the application of the disposing power. This is a man. That is a savage. The names justify differences in treatment.

At the same time that speech delivers Man from appetite and fear, domesticating the fear of death and regularizing the ubiquitous and contingent violence of nature, it also exposes Man to distinctively human vices. Only men lie or declare their will to be otherwise than it is. Only men make false promises or promises they are unable to keep. While nature "hath armed living creatures, some with teeth, some with horns, and some with hands, to grieve an enemy," only men use words to manage, manipulate, torment, or condemn one another, either as a substitute for physical violence or by decreeing the *right* to violence.[31] Words themselves become objects upon which men act. Words, no less than a luscious fruit or a man with a knife, stimulate appetite and fear. Power consists in owning the words of command and in being able to employ words to make others act in accordance with one's own will. The vices of speech—intimidation, dishonesty, hypocrisy, dissembling—provide effective strategies in the exercise of that power.

Speech distinguishes Man from other creatures, not only because it makes possible the voluntary will and the promise of the covenant that will secure peace but also because it provides the material infrastructure for the signs of power. Titles, honors, offices, and reputation serve as "so many signs of favour in the Common-wealth; which favour is Power."[32] Power resides in the rules about who can say what to whom and who has the power of decree over others. The master's power consists in his right to a certain mode of speech: the command. By the sovereign's right to pronounce judgment over all and to decree what will be, he fixes "the publique rate of the worth of . . . men." He who controls the power of names controls the disposition of men.

A man may misuse words, misapplying names or combining them badly, so that he deceives himself. He may employ them so that nothing is conceived in them. The privilege of words brings with it the "priviledge of Absurdity; to which no living creature is subject, but man onely."[33] The men most susceptible to this vice are those "that professe Philosophy." Their words may be so disconnected from sensuous experience as not to be about anything real.

This danger of abstraction manifests itself in the contemporary discourse of human rights. The Universal Declaration of Human Rights (La declaration universelle des droits de l'homme) articulates an abstract concept of the human person and abstract rights of equality, while, in many of its signatory states, these rights do not exist or are enjoyed only by a privileged class. Article 21, for example, states that "everyone has the right of equal access to public service in his [sic] country," but, in many states, women and particular races or ethnic groups are either prohibited from participating in the institutions that govern their lives or are so dramatically underrepresented as to suggest some structural, rather than accidental, inequity. If, as Article 17 insists, "no one should be arbitrarily deprived of his [sic] property," then why are indigenous farmers regularly displaced in many of the signatory countries? If, as Article 3 proclaims, everyone has "the right to the security of his [sic] person," then why are individuals in many signatory states subject to surveillance, isolation, or imprisonment without due process? How does this right assure the "security of a [woman's] person" if the signatory state can intervene in her most intimate decisions about reproduction? If, as Article 16 decrees, men and women have the right to marry without limitation due to race, nationality, or religion; if men and women are entitled to equal rights as to marriage, during marriage, and at its dissolution; and if marriage depends on the free consent of the intending spouses, then why are women in many signatory states murdered for attempting to marry outside their ethnic group, denied divorce or equal property rights, or married without their consent? Does the document's emphasis on civil rights in the public sphere and its valorization of the family as the "natural and fundamental group unit of society" not ignore the violence and subjection that take place within the family in many signatory states?

These declarations of abstract rights that belong only to an abstract "person" disregard the specificities of experience that actually determine human life. In doing so, such declarations advance speculative concepts of "equality" and "dignity" that hide the real structural inequities in which actual human beings live. Power is exercised through the discourse of human rights itself, and human rights and human rights law may be a "mask" for injustice and an "instrument for domination" in its own right.[34]

The strategy of abstraction that belongs to the discourse of rights divests *the right* of its essential character as a *claim* or *command*. On whom do these rights make a claim? On whom does the obligation fall to deliver what is promised in them? Everyone and no one. These abstract rights depend on Man's consent and are established according to the test of reason. As Onora O'Neill has argued, rights are empty "until we know who has what obligation to do what for whom under which circumstances."[35] Unless the powerful, those capable of acting, are convinced of their obligation, the declaration of rights offers a sanitizing rhetoric instead of the right.

The power of abstraction that distinguishes men among all other living creatures provides the strategy whereby Man installs himself as the figure of the human.[36] Man speaks in and for the human, whose status as the genus has been clarified and articulated through the exclusion of women, children, "the savages of the Americas," the poor (who are always dishonorable), and men who lack "self-reliance" or the passion for power. Absent from the "little Monarchy of the family," women appear whenever it is a question of sexual rights. Hobbes insists that it is a greater crime to violate the chastity of a married woman than of an unmarried woman, a claim that can only be founded on an interpretation of the offense as a violation of the husband's property rights.[37] Women appear to be used and disposed of as the property of men.

Women also serve as a foil for the display of Man's properties or what is proper to Man. Hobbes repeatedly insists on the necessity that a man must think for himself, rather than relying on the opinions of "Schoolmen" or other authorities. Women, like children, are given to "weeping" because they are incapable of this distinctively human self-reliance (chapter 6, 43). Unable to engage in the abstract reasoning that makes a man master of his own experience, women are inclined toward "dejection," "causeless fears," and "Melancholy" (chapter 8, 54). Hobbes approvingly relates the story of a "Graecian City" in which the "young Maidens" were seized by a madness that "caused many of them to hang themselves." The magistrates, supposing that the maidens still regarded their honor if not their lives, gave an order to "strip such as so hang'd themselves, and let them hang out naked" (chapter 8, 56). Apparently, this stopped the hangings, though it is not clear, as Hobbes asserts, that it "cured the madnesse" or ended the maidens' suffering.

More subtly, Hobbes introduces into the abstraction Man those differences among men that will justify social inequity and hierarchies of power. Differences in power and wealth marked the fictive moment of consent from the very beginning and thereby disfigured the Covenant, Peace, and Sovereign Power. The covenant transforms these inequities into rights, sustaining them by the threat of violence displayed in the subtle signs of the system of sovereign power. "The *Value,* or Worth of a man, is as of all other things, his Price, that is to say so much as would be given for the use of his Power" (chapter 10, 63). Like any commodity, a man's value is determined by the price he can command in the market. Whatever he may think of himself, his value depends on the estimation of others, on what they will pay for his favor or service, as well as on the power that he exerts over others. "Riches, are honourable for they are Power. Poverty, Dishonourable" (chapter 10, 66). Similarly, to be born of "conspicuous" parents is honorable, because they are more likely to be able to obtain the aid of powerful relations and friends. To descend from "obscure Parentage" is dishonorable. "Dominion and victory" are honorable; "Servitude," whether out of need or fear, is dishonorable.

Worth or honor derives from power: "Honourable is whatsoever possession, action, or quality, is an argument and signe of Power" (chapter 10, 65). Power consists in the "means, to obtain some future apparent Good" (62). Strength is Power, as is Beauty insofar as it "recommendeth men to the favour of women and strangers" (63). Friends and Reputation are Power insofar as they encourage others to adhere to a man's will. "Couvetousness of great Riches, and ambition of great Honours" are signs of power (66). Power, like a heavy stone set in motion, gathering speed, feeds upon itself. Power begets more power and an increased ambition or desire for power (chapter 5, 35). The "general inclination of all mankind, [is] a perpetuall and restless desire of Power after power, that ceaseth only in Death." Man cannot be confident in the power that he has "without the acquisition of more" (chapter 11, 72).

Differences in "Wit" derive from differences in the "desire of Power" (chapter 13, 53). A man who has no great passion for power will be limited both in imagination and judgment, for the desire to obtain the goods that power makes accessible provides the chief impetus for these faculties. "Thoughts are to the Desires, as Scouts, and Spies, to range abroad, and find the way to the things

Desired" (chapter 13, 53). A man who lacks a robust passion for power may be deficient in his desire for the satisfying goods, but he will lack as well the motivation to imagine and think. Some men, content to behave like animals, acting on the last appetite, are less capable and less interested than others in discerning cause and effect, general rules, and the abstract concepts that make it possible to govern fields of particulars.

Successful men are like good sporting dogs: they are motivated by a passion for "Ranging"; hunters, they traverse a field of evidence on the move in search of their prey. Just as the hounds might track a fox or deer and the spaniel a duck or other fowl, a man with an appetite for honor thinks foremost on "the next means of attaining it." Honor, as a form of power, amplifies itself by the logic of the *always more.* "And this the Latins call *sagacitas,* SAGACITY, and we may call it hunting or tracing, as dogs trace the beast by the smell, and men hunt them by their footsteps; or as men hunt after riches, place, or knowledge."[38] Motivated by an appetite for power, Man lives in search of it.

Philosophers hunt down those names and principles that will facilitate Man's dual aim of satisfying appetite and eliminating threat. General names enable Man to position himself as the custodian of other living creatures: women, children, savages, other animals, nature, Earth. General names make it possible to treat actual humanbodies as *instances of a class.* Specific humanbodies become disposable subjects—treated, incarcerated, punished, disciplined, motivated, indoctrinated—*as members of this class.* A humanbody who belongs to one of Man's excluded classes often finds that a proper name exerts little power compared to the power of disposition exercised through the general name of membership in this class.

Hobbes insists that "all men by nature reason alike,"[39] eliding the specific differences and identities that determine human life. At the same time, he insinuates into Man, the generic figure of the human, quantitative and qualitative differences in passion and in the capacity for abstraction that produce rules of mastery and obedience as well as the justification for differences in power and wealth. The names of exclusion and the proprieties of *right* relegate some to rule and others to obey. Those who, from a lack of passion more than ability, do not develop the powers of speech and abstract thought "are in this point like children, that having no thought of generation, are made believe by the women, that their brothers and sisters are not born, but found in the garden."[40] Their credulity reflects not only their deficiency in discerning general principles of cause and effect but also their lack of power and their destiny to serve others more powerful than themselves. They may exhibit the prudence of animals, but they are incapable of science or knowledge of principles. A man may be dexterous in handling arms, but unless he knows the *science* of fencing, all the possible ways by which to attack his opponent and all the possible moves for his defense, his dexterity will prove a weak power against the man who possesses both that power and its principles.[41] The man of science imagines the others' parries and thrusts before they happen according to the possibilities of fencing itself. His actions are not, like those of the animals, based on experience and sense, merely prudential; rather, they anticipate and respond to an array of possible futures. To dexterity and experience, the man of science adds the power to project and act on an image of the future by imposing names and rules on nature itself.

Thoughts move a man's body. They may move him to create in words an image of the future that moves the bodies of other men. A man, Hobbes, for example, understandably shaken by the terror of civil war, recreates nature in an image as that war.

Against the awesome terror of the fear of death, he pits the Colossus of the "Artificial Person," whose measure in the signs of power called *civil* or *political life* can only be approached by "*Leviathan*," the largest creature ever to live on earth or a sea monster so vast and fabulous that it appears only when the gods do. Sticking fast to the instinct of self-preservation as the motive force of life, Hobbes capitalizes on the bet that some will acquiesce out of the fear of death, and that some, for lack of that peculiar collaboration between passion and thought that marks the successful man, will serve, while others command. He installs an image of the future that does not so much replace might by right, but joins right to might in the legitimation of social inequity and hierarchies of power, putting in place a system of names and associated principles that will play an essential authorizing role in Man's legalized servitude and legitimate violence.

Names and other images—a great whale, a sovereign man, a frontispiece—may move men to action: to read the book, to discuss and agree on its truth, to refer to it in elaborating legal systems and justifications of state policy, to read it still centuries later, something that *must be read*, because we live by its names and myths.

The whale resurfaces. Ahab gives the command.

ROUSSEAU AND HEGEL: CUSTOMS, CODES, AND THE GENDER DIVISION OF LABOR

When the meal went on too long and fine weather called me, I could not wait till the others had finished, and leaving them at table I would make my escape and install myself all alone in a boat, which I would row out into the middle of the lake when it was calm; and there, stretching out full-length in the boat and turning my eyes skyward, I let myself float and drift wherever the water took me, often for several hours on end, plunged in a host of vague yet delightful reveries . . . infinitely to be preferred to all that I had found most sweet in the so-called pleasures of life.

    —JEAN-JACQUES ROUSSEAU, *REVERIES OF A SOLITARY WALKER* (1778)

Woman, honor the head of your house. It is he who works for you, who wins your bread, who feeds you. This is man.

    —JEAN-JACQUES ROUSSEAU, *EMILE; OR, ON EDUCATION* (1762)

Since the community only gets an existence through its interference with the happiness of the Family, and by dissolving self-consciousness into the universal, it creates for itself in what it suppresses and what is at the same time essential to it an internal enemy—womankind in general.

    —G. W. F. HEGEL, *PHENOMENOLOGY OF SPIRIT* (1807)

At sea in a frail craft, threatened by a massive storm, an ocean of chaos stretching to the horizon, Man teeters on the edge of life. The colossus rises to meet his disaster. Unleashing an awesome power of distinction and definition, *Leviathan* secures Man, rewriting nature as life under sovereign power.

Rousseau's texts offer a decided change of weather and a very different atmosphere and landscape. Their narrator wanders a rustic garden path on a bright morning or sips coffee in a charming inn as the evening wanes. We are no longer on the battlefield or the open sea. Rowing on a *calm lake,* the narrator spends several hours afloat and adrift, stretched out in the boat, looking up at the sky, lost in "delightful reveries," until he notices the orange and pink horizon of the setting sun.[42] The concepts of natural right, transfer of right, sovereignty, property, and law that Hobbes articulates, like Adam naming the animals, are for Rousseau ready-made cultural artifacts, ready to hand and ready to be rehearsed. They already inform life, but imperfectly due to error or deception. The task is not so much to secure peace against an indefinite state of war as it is to discern the sincerity or hypocrisy of the law and the hierarchies of power.

For the most part, Rousseau restages Hobbes' account of the transition from natural life to civil society. Man's solitary life in nature might be happy, but, when he comes in contact with other men, envy and competition erupt.[43] Men are haunted by a "dark propensity to harm each other."[44] An "original covenant" subordinating liberty to law is necessary to regulate violence and ownership.[45] Each man "alienates" his will and right, transferring it to the whole to create the general will or sovereign power. As an "unconditional" alienation performed by each man, the covenant creates equality among men, transforming "natural" equality into a "moral" or "legal" equality.[46] Each man is said to make the pledge "under the same conditions," and the transfer of his right to the general will is reciprocated when the general will acts through its institutions on his behalf.

Rousseau emphasizes that, in what appears to be a renunciation, Man actually turns a profit. An owner is not deprived of his goods under the social contract; rather, a man's possessions are restored to him as *property.* Every owner is a "trustee" of sovereign power. What before he merely possessed on his own, he now owns by right of sovereign power; what is alienated in the moment of the contract returns with an added value. As a result of the social contract, men "have profitably exchanged an uncertain and precarious life for a better and more secure one."[47] If the covenant secures possession as property, possession guaranteed by sovereign power, then the contract will always have been between owners or men of property. The renunciation only makes a profit if what is renounced is recovered and held more securely. Thus "each man recovers the equivalent of everything he loses, and in the bargain he acquires more power to preserve what he has."[48]

Either the contract redistributes the wealth accumulated by might in the state of nature or it reinforces these inequities of wealth by covering them with law. The absolute alienation of each man from his goods and person and his aggregation in the body politic will not produce equality if what has been alienated is always recovered with a profit. The contract cannot be reciprocal, as the owner's relation to the general will cannot be the same as the poor man's: given what is to be alienated and returned in each case, the owner receives a much larger return on his risk. His possessions have become property, protected under the law of the sovereign. The poor man is still poor, but now not as a matter of the accidents of might but as a matter of *right*. The rhetorical stage is now set for all those industrial and postindustrial discourses on the reasons for poverty and the (un)deserving poor. The rhetoric of rights established by the contract cannot be detached from these structural inequalities.[49] The right to property legitimates them.

This impossible contract, Rousseau breezily concedes, never took place, "but, though perhaps never formally stated, [its articles] are everywhere the same, everywhere tacitly admitted and recognized."[50] Everywhere and nowhere. The mythical contract performs an illusory renunciation in order to install a fiction of equality that will legitimate inequities of wealth and power. "The figure of the social contract obscures the fact of the entanglement of rights discourse with power relations since it leads one to see rights both as the spontaneous product of an unforced consensus and as equally beneficial for all rights bearers."[51] The fiction of consent hides the grafting of right onto what might has already secured for itself.

Rousseau is not unaware of the problem. He insists that the social contract will ameliorate the inequities in liberty and wealth that arise from natural inequities in strength and intelligence, but the profit-making renunciation makes no opportunity for any redistribution of goods or power. In a footnote he admits that under "bad government" equality may be an "illusion." Under bad government the doctrine of equality "serves only to keep the poor in their wretchedness and sustain the rich in their usurpation."[52] Law serves wealth: "In truth, laws are always useful to those with possessions and harmful to those who have nothing." Rousseau infers that "the social state is useful to men only when all possess something and none has too much."[53]

Beyond this marginal advisory against the ill effects on the general will of excessive economic inequity, the narrative of the contract, the renunciation or alienation that creates the general will, transforms the wealth and power held by might into property protected by law. Man's transference of the right to dispose of all property to sovereign power does not undo ownership. The contract actually secures ownership by transforming possession into property *held by right*, against which others can now *make no claim*. Rousseau cautions against extreme economic inequity, while exempting the concept of equality from the requirement that power and wealth be "the same for all."[54] While the rich should learn "moderation in goods and influence," the poor must learn "moderation in avarice and covetousness." They should learn to want less.

Life and death set the limits of inequity: "No citizen shall be rich enough to buy another and none so poor as to be forced to sell himself."[55] Certainly, such buying and selling occurred in Rousseau's own time, just as it does in ours. Slavery, indentured servitude, and prostitution all still flourish today. In addition, new medical technologies have created markets in organs and wombs. Feminist bioethicists argue in support of the poor Indian woman's "right" to sell her eggs or womb.[56] In the discourse of rights, the body belongs to property and can be disposed of like other forms of property. Some people are so poor they have nothing left to market but themselves. Rousseau argues against such selling and buying not because it is wrong in itself, but because it causes "sectionalism" and undermines the cohesion of the state. Curb the excesses of wealth just enough not to offend; give the poor just enough to keep them complacent. Having confessed earlier that the law always favors the wealthy and powerful, Rousseau insists that the "force of legislation ought always be to preserve [equality]," but only so much equality as is necessary to the stability of the state.[57]

Like Hobbes, Rousseau employs the conceit of an "Artificial Person" to describe sovereignty or the general will. Like the swarm of bees, the body politic comprises a multitude of members whose cohesion depends on the regulatory power of a general will. Just as a man can control his own arms and legs, so too the social contract gives the "body politic an absolute power over all its members."[58] Sovereignty names that power of the general will. Rousseau distinguishes sovereignty, or the legislative power, from government, or the executive power invested in the prince. While the prince is the "brain" of the body politic that sets its members in motion, the legislative power is its heart. A man may live as an imbecile, but if his heart stops he is dead.[59] Sovereignty, the power to decree law, is the lifeblood of the body politic.

Unfortunately, the body politic suffers a congenital defect. "Just as the particular will acts unceasingly against the general will, so does the government continually exert itself against the sovereign."[60] The health of the body politic depends on an identity of the prince's will with that of the sovereign power or general will. Three tendencies undermine that identity and act on the body politic like "old age and death": first, the tendency of the prince to pursue aims that are personal rather than general; second, the tendency of the government to identify itself with his aims; and third, the tendency of the government to become an aim in its own right and to establish itself as an end distinct from sovereignty or the general will. Government should mediate between sovereignty and the people, translating the general will into actual policies and practices, but its tendency is to serve the prince or itself. As a result, the citizen is less sovereign and more subject. It is less likely that his interests will coincide with the government's aims, and more likely that the former will be sacrificed to the latter.

In the myth of contract, citizens have also sacrificed their right to life by transferring it to the sovereign and the executive authority of the prince. The purpose of the contract was the preservation of the members who were party to it. Each one agreed to cede his *liberty to use violence* to secure his ends by investing the *right to violence* in the prince who will protect each and all. If the prince deems the death of a citizen necessary to the security of the state, then "he should die." The contract transforms the life of the citizen, so that it is "no longer the bounty of nature but a gift he has received conditionally from the state."[61] This subjection of life to the prince as the executor of sovereignty exposes life to strategic management, opening the way for government to dispose of life so as to serve its own ends more efficiently. The power to put to death authorizes the optimal utilization of life. This will take many forms, from conscription into the military to the regulation of labor and consumption in markets.

While Hobbes defined citizenship, Rousseau concentrates on how citizenship is to be produced. Hobbes hardly mentions education, except to imply that it will be limited to the very small class of persons who are capable of science. In

1762, the same year as the publication of *The Social Contract*, Rousseau publishes a second much longer text devoted entirely to the theory and practice of educating Man, the man of reason, the citizen.

Like Hobbes, Rousseau limits education by class and race. Education does not address the fixity of the class structure by introducing mobility. "The poor man does not need to be educated. His station gives him a compulsory education."[62] Experience teaches the poor all they need to know: being poor teaches you how to be poor. Emile, the narrator's chosen pupil, is taught not to give money to the poor, as "they usually employ it badly."[63] He is taught instead to share their labor enough to understand it and to supply them with the means of their own labor and comfort: a cow, a plow, or a new roof. Man's role with respect to the poor is that of "benefactor," whose aim is to provide the poor with the means to make the best of their poverty, not to transcend it.

Like Hobbes, Rousseau limits education to Anglo-Europeans as opposed to "savages." Rousseau may refer to an admirable savage uncorrupted by the vanity and hypocrisy of Anglo-European culture, but that savage is not capable of the same rational life as Man. In principle, he cannot join the community of men who all "reason alike." "Neither the Negroes, nor the Laplanders have the sense of the Europeans."[64] Rousseau speculates that, in their extreme climates, the "organization of the brain is less perfect." Some bodies are congenitally unsuited for the rational program that produces Man.

Rousseau grafts onto Hobbes' exclusions a rhetoric of health and sickness, prefiguring biopower and the complicity of medicine in disciplining race and sex. Starting from the chaos of civil war, Hobbes aims to replace violence with security. Starting from the corruption of human nature by bad government and the vain hypocrisy of society, Rousseau prescribes a new regimen of government and education to restore the health and honesty of Man.

In choosing the pupil who will benefit from his educational experiment, the narrator of *Emile* rejects any "sickly or ill-constituted child." While a father is obliged to love and care for all his children, whatever their condition, caring for a "sickly or "crippled" child would transform the "governor" into a "male nurse." The narrator of *Emile* will not waste his time "caring for a useless life."[65] The pupil must be of the right nature and have the right capacities to take advantage of the governor's knowledge and pedagogy.

A male child remains under the dominion of the "little Monarch" only until he reaches his majority and becomes a "little Monarch" in his own right. The pupil's whole education tends toward this independence. Women, like the poor, savages, and the chronically ill or disabled, cannot be educated for autonomous life. While males progress from childhood to manhood, developing rationality and distinguishing themselves one from the other, women, like eunuchs, "are always big children" (211).

While Hobbes installs Man as the "little Monarch" of the family, Rousseau maps in detail the "small fatherland which is the family" (363). From the diet of nursing mothers and household hygiene to the introduction of language and science, the cultivation of virtues and manners, and the inculcation of the responsibilities of citizenship, Rousseau ties the abstractions of right and contract to the smallest quotidian detail. Medicine, nutrition, regimes of exercise, courses of instruction, codes of belief, and norms of behavior comprise an extensive apparatus for the transformation of the man of nature into the citizen Man. An ancillary apparatus provides for the production of his wife, who "completes" him.

Men and women must be educated differently, according to their different destinies. Men are formed by the "order of nature" to reason, women to "obey" and to "please" (370, see also 407). Science or the "quest for abstract and speculative truth" should not be part of women's education, "for everything that tends to generalize ideas, is not within the competence of women" (386). Rousseau prescribes for women practices of "habitual constraint" that will ensure women's "docility." Girls may be allowed to play and frolic, but "do not allow for a single instant in their lives that they no longer know any restraint. Accustom them to being interrupted in the midst of their games and brought back to other cares without grumbling" (370). This restraint is essential for two reasons. First, "almost from infancy women are on the defensive and entrusted with a treasure that is difficult to protect" (397). The dangers to which a young girl is exposed are evident in the narrator / governor's own imagination: "When someone sees her, he says, 'Here is a modest, temperate girl.' But so long as he stays near her, his eyes and his heart roam over her whole person without his being able to take them away; and one would say that all this very simple attire was put on only to be taken off piece by piece by the imagination" (394). Habits of self-control and an instinctive check on gaiety and frivolity will serve to protect a woman's modesty and reputation from the disrobing eyes of men. Rousseau declares a woman responsible not only for being faithful but also for acting so as to make it possible for her husband to believe that she is faithful (361). She is responsible not just for his sexual pleasure but also for his jealousy or peace of mind.

Second, the application to girls of a regimen of "habitual constraint" will prepare them "to learn early to endure even injustice and to bear a husband's wrongs without complaining" (370, see also 396). Women's duties prohibit her from seeking justice; her personal claim is sacrificed to the "moral person" that she forms with her husband.[66] As a wife's responsibility includes the duty to "make herself loved and honored," the victim of domestic abuse may be responsible for her own fate. Even an "insensitive and barbarous man" will be civilized by the presence of a virtuous and comely young girl (390). Rousseau advises wives to substitute careful counsel for churlish complaint.

While Rousseau repeatedly insists that a woman's destiny is to obey and to submit to the men who are responsible for her, he just as regularly ascribes to her a certain indirect mastery. She reigns in an "empire of gentleness" (408, see also 387). Through "caresses" and "tears," she manages her husband, "getting herself commanded to do what she wants to do." It is her responsibility to ensure the happiness of both by joining her sentiment to his reason. Lovable and desirable, she can motivate a man to right action, to both virtue and productivity. She can move the miser to charity, the libertine to chastity, and the glutton to moderation. Women are the "natural judges of men's merit" (390, see also 398). While nature requires her submission to Man, woman retains an invisible authority by working the levers of a man's heart. She practices an "experimental morality," based on intuition and experience, rather than law (387). Her task is to learn to please a man so as to influence him for the better. "Thus, the whole education of women ought to relate to men" (365). While modesty, passivity, and submission should be cultivated in young girls, women should be taught to manage men through a combination of sexual gratification and the threat of unpleasant scenes. She must not be a "coquette," but "at once decent, lovable, and self-controlled." If she develops her natural ability to "read men's hearts," she will know how to influence men to act according to her own aims. She who is both loved and esteemed "sends her lovers with a nod to the end of the world, to combat, to glory, to death, to anything she pleases" (393). The happiness of the marriage and of the two partners, as well as her husband's success, depends upon her, even as she is denied any real agency, any agency not corrupted from the start by deception all around.

Rousseau repeatedly denounces women who champion political rights for women, just as he disdains women who undertake intellectual work. These "literary maidens" should remain maidens, as "sensible men" would not have them. Women who seek rights in the political sphere want to have their rights and Man's. They undermine the natural social divisions of the two sexes (409, see also 364). These women are unnatural or antinatural. In Rousseau's theme of corruption lurks a harmful woman denatured by a bad education. This discourse begins to join diagnoses of what is natural and healthy to the state's interest in shaping citizens to be productive members of the body politic. Education, medicine, and government participate mutually in the maintenance of sexual propriety and the productivity of property.

Mary Wollstonecraft anticipates Nietzsche, Simone de Beauvoir, and Foucault in arguing that women are made, not born.[67] Directing her remarks largely against Rousseau, Wollstonecraft argues that a woman's limitations reflect not her nature but the educational program to which she has been subjected. If she is weak, silly, and given to frivolous pursuits, it is because she has been cultivated to be so. Wollstonecraft deems Rousseau's anecdotal proofs that girls are *naturally* weak or concerned with personal appearance or given to playing with dolls as "below contempt." Girls enjoy and benefit from the same regimens of exercise and science in the same ways that boys do. Girls who are educated well will be as women at least as rational as men. The ideology advanced by Rousseau, that the destiny of woman is to please and be subject to Man, installs "this brutal desire of self-preservation [as] the grand spring of all her actions" (151). An education that cultivates delicacy, modesty, simplicity, and a concern with appearances tends to produce the weak mind and body that Rousseau ascribes to women.

Wollstonecraft also anticipates contemporary commentators who argue that improving women's education improves the quality of life for the whole community: "Till women are more rationally educated, the progress of human virtue and improvement in knowledge must receive continual check" (107). Women need both physical strength and a good education to be prepared to take care of their families and themselves, but the idea that a woman's fate is determined by her attractiveness to men is the "iron bed of fate, to fit which her character should be stretched or contracted, regardless of all moral or physical distinctions" (151). Wollstonecraft rails against Rousseau and other writers on the education of women for tending to "degrade one half of the human species, and render women pleasing at the expense of every solid virtue" (87). Women can be "really virtuous and useful" only when they are physically robust, educated, and economically independent.

Wollstonecraft's analysis calls into question both the norms of sexual propriety and the laws of property. Women in many countries that are signatories to international declarations of rights continue to be "subjected by ignorance to their sensations," "denied all political privileges," taught that the "mighty business of female life is to please," and "restrained from entering into more important concerns by political and civil oppression" (272–73). Even where women appear to have political rights, it is usual for them to be dramatically underrepresented in decision making and leadership in nearly every arena. Even if they are not sold in marriage or servitude, as in some tribal cultures, women in high-income countries find their bodies used in marketing or find themselves determined by their sexuality and marriage status or the objects of unwanted attention in the workplace or at home. Decades of research indicate the subtle ways that girls are tracked into the "helping" or "serving" professions. In the United States, women appeared to fare better than men after the Great Recession, until analysts realized that increases in employment were mainly at the lowest wages or part time, positions that tend to be held by women more frequently than by men.

Wollstonecraft's polemic of 1792 addresses problems that persist today, and it anticipates the idea that women's rights are *human* rights. Like Luce Irigaray, Wollstonecraft realizes that *equal* rights for women will not quite address the problem, as women "may have different duties to fulfill." As women's duties "are *human* duties," thinking from them may have a universal effect, changing the narrative of ethics and extending the principles of moral philosophy.[68] Women must be educated to take their place as participating citizens of the civil and political community, both because justice requires it and because this inclusion improves the life of the whole community. By extending civil and political rights to women and by grafting "women's duties" onto man's, Wollstonecraft creates a new hybrid right that transgresses property and sexual propriety to promote the generativity of women.

In Rousseau's canonical analysis, however, women enjoy only the "right to be weak." Having admonished girls not to play the coquette and having emphasized the necessity of "honesty," "purity," and "trust," both to a woman's character and in her relationships, Rousseau nonetheless prescribes for the wife a strategy of dissimulation. She is to appear weak, while invisibly managing her husband's affections and pleasure to manipulate him into doing what she wants. Indeed, she often *pretends* to be weak. As a "shrewd precaution," women affect delicacy to "prepare in advance excuses . . . in case of need."[69] Rousseau prescribes for women the very hypocrisy and vanity he identifies as the nidus of all social ills and the reason men are "in chains." Wollstonecraft demonstrates how feigned weakness becomes real weakness both in women and in the civil and political community.

By the time Hegel publishes the *Phenomenology of Spirit* in 1807, the figures of Man and woman are well articulated and ready to hand. The infrastructures of education, public health, labor, and commerce that will regulate these identities have already permeated most domains of life. Industrialization and urbanization already call for the scientific management of populations to protect public health and increase efficiency and productivity. Bureaucracy will survey and administer life in all its registers.

Hegel, like Hobbes and Rousseau, offers a mythological account of the origin of society in which contact between men in the state of nature inevitably produces a "struggle unto death." He who risks life absolutely and prevails in the fight becomes the master; he who acquiesces in the fight out of the fear of death becomes the slave. History unfolds from this relation, as the slave, through his labor and discipline, regains his freedom in the modern nation-state. States are founded on agriculture and marriage. Agriculture introduces private property. Marriage transforms private need into care for the family and possession into family property.[70] Together they ensure "security, consolidation, lasting satisfaction of need." Rather than speculate a mythical moment of contract, Hegel focuses on the way in which a concrete general will embodied in a nation-state arises out of private property and the family. In his account, as in Hobbes' and Rousseau's, human society emerges out of the fear of death, and men form a community of mutual recognition or a nation of laws only in order to address the violent competition and insecurity to which they are otherwise subject. While

Rousseau details microtechniques of power for the education and discipline of bodies—hygiene, exercise, manners, habit—Hegel focuses on the macroinstitutions that sustain Man's hegemony—the family, the state, and the gender division of labor.

The family is the "element of the Nation." As birds live in the element of air and fish live in water, so too the citizen lives in a family. As the material element of the state, the family supplies its labor and its future. The brother's destiny is to leave the family behind so that he can participate in the "universal" domains of politics, science, and philosophy; the sister's is to become a wife. She will care for the body and blood, bearing children and burying the dead, so that Man may be free for his discursive pursuits.

Just as human life depends biologically on sexual difference, so too its ethical life is organized around the difference between Man and woman. Man will participate in the self-conscious, self-legislating collectives of science and politics, while woman will preserve the unconscious domain of blood relationship. While men act in the world to create the material infrastructures that would actually sustain mutual recognition among them, women remain isolated in the family. Deprived of real opportunities for solidarity, living in a culture of possibilities lethal to female solidarities, only vicariously through her brother does she glimpse an image of citizenship.

Hegel's analysis addresses a real problem: the lack of material infrastructures for the integration of work and family. For millennia, human beings have solved this problem through the gender division of labor. When women enter into public domains of work, Hegel argues, they put society itself in danger.[71] Contemporary experience confirms his analysis. As women have entered the public workforce, child care and the care of the sick and aged have become social issues. The obesity epidemic in the United States is directly related to a sharp decrease in home cooking.[72] Articles and books abound advising women on how to "have it all" or on the wisdom of not having it all. Data indicate that women who work outside the home still carry an overwhelming share of the burden of work in the home.[73] Young educated women report a disinclination to work due to the suffering they have observed in their mothers as they tried to manage work and family, giving up the struggle before it has even begun.[74] The persistent intensity of debates around work and family and woman's place reflect the unsustainable lack of infrastructures for integrating work and family, for sustaining both participation in the public sphere and the generativity of the body.

The gender division of labor depends on women's status as property and on the enforcement of sexual propriety. It efficiently solves the problem of how to serve the public worlds of science, politics, and philosophy while also sustaining the body of the family. Today men remain overrepresented in the counsels that determine the future. Women remain economically dependent on men and earn less for their labor. Around the globe, economic and cultural forces impose an image of women as the object of male desire. Laws, codes, and institutions reinforce narratives of identity for women that focus on the value of a woman's virginity and the moment when it is given away / sold to a man. Her intimate generativity is given / sold, with all that this implies in terms of a life of caring for others, in exchange for being "endowed with all his worldly goods." He goes to work, while she sustains generativity. She feeds and cares for life, for the growth of children, for the comfort of aging parents, or for the relief of the sick; she tends the body of the man who works too.

The forces reinforcing these differentiated identities deploy from multiple directions: dress codes, patterns of surveillance, restrictions on mobility and association, as well as regimens of discipline, obedience, and punishment. Massive economic forces—from the dowry or bride price in South Asia to the Long Island wedding industry—aggressively deploy this narrative. It will not be easy to dislodge such an effective apparatus for addressing the vital and necessary need to sustain both public enterprise and the intimate life of the family. The controlling themes of political philosophy—the discontinuity of natural and civil life, the inherently violent nature of Man, the necessity for some form of sovereignty or mastery to keep that nature in check, the substitution of right for might, the inevitability of social inequity, the status of women as property, and the invisibility of women in the public arenas where decisions about the community's future are made—work together to sustain and authorize this system.

Abstract rights cannot be disentangled from the right to property, nor from the norms of sexual and racial identity that serve hierarchies of power and wealth. The discourse of rights is complicit with biopower, with the institutions, codes, and practices that enforce sexual propriety and maximize the productivity of generative bodies.

2

Capitalized Bodies

BIOETHICS, BIOPOWER, AND THE
PRACTICE OF FREEDOM

For millennia, man remained what he was for Aristotle: a living animal with the additional capacity for a political existence; modern man is an animal whose politics places his existence as a living being in question.

—MICHEL FOUCAULT, *THE HISTORY OF SEXUALITY*, VOL. 1 (1976)

For the same reason that they have—or ought to have—little freedom, they tend to excess in the freedom that is left to them. Extreme in everything, they indulge themselves in their games with even more intensity than boys do. . . . Do not deprive them of gaiety, laughter, noise, and frolicsome games, but prevent them from getting their fill of one in order to run to another: do not allow for a single instant in their lives that they no longer know any restraint. Accustom them to being interrupted in the midst of their games and brought back to other cares without grumbling.

—JEAN-JACQUES ROUSSEAU, *EMILE* (1762)

Stem cell research, genetic testing, cloning: progress in the life sciences is giving human beings new power to improve our health and control the development processes of all living species.

—UNESCO BIOETHICS SECTION WEBSITE (2013)

Ashamed of their incompleteness, human beings have turned themselves into experimental beings.

—JEAN BAUDRILLARD, *THE AGONY OF POWER* (2005)

IN ROUSSEAU'S DESCRIPTION, the "frolicking" of the blooming young girls—perhaps, they are picking crocus and narcissus in a floriferous meadow—displays a threatening "intensity" that must be carefully regulated and restrained.[1] They suffer from an "excess" of vivacity and must be tamed, not only to avoid any danger to the supreme value of their chastity and reputation but also to train them for their submissive, supporting role later on. Perhaps philosophers have always wanted to "control the development processes of all living species." The UNESCO definition of bioethics refers to control at the biological level, but institutions, codes, laws, and practices have long been in place to manage the development of human life and to turn the plasticity of the human animal toward certain identities: Man of reason, citizen, worker, wife. Like the regimens, disciplines, and instructions prescribed by Rousseau in *Emile,* these infrastructures of life and identity are pervasive, regulating every dimension of experience: hygiene, physical mobility, sexuality, work, even child's play. Here, among the warm bodies of a gaggle of girls, the abstract names of philosophy find a carnal realization.

Rousseau's example already exhibits the mature features of a *disciplinary power* that will prove to be the mode of transition between sovereign power and biopower:

- Human life becomes an object of scientific study based on the difference between the normal and the pathological.
- Knowledge becomes the property of experts. This expert knowledge provides the basis for development plans to train individuals into their proper identity, particularly into sexual propriety.
- These plans require extensive surveillance and evaluation.
- This training or taming involves more or less violent interventions into bodily integrity, including the use of force, the infliction of pain or pleasure, and the limitation of physical mobility.
- This training or taming aims to inculcate the proper identity so that the individual becomes self-policing and there is no need for any external discipline.

By enjoining their governesses never to let the young girls feel on their own or at liberty, Rousseau means to erect internal restraints, replacing the girls' effusive vivacity with obedience and care. The girls are not merely to be restrained but also *made otherwise* as required by the identity to which their sex destines them.[2]

While Rousseau writes of the intimate relation of tutor and student, the regimens and disciplines of the "governor" were already being disseminated in state-sanctioned institutions and agencies such as schools, hospitals, public health services, police forces, and in government policy. By the beginning of the nineteenth century, virtually every area of human life had come under some kind of scrutiny involving a collusion of science and the state. The scientific study of sexuality, for example, gave rise to intense surveillance of childhood sexuality. Parents were encouraged to discover their child in the act of masturbation. This was prima facie evidence of disease, so that the result of the parents' observation was their own displacement as the authority in the child's life by the experts and the experts' knowledge of how to extinguish this pathological behavior.[3] From the mid-eighteenth century on, human life became something to be managed by scientific theory and state policy.

Increasingly, the aim of these interventions has been to regulate the bodies of individuals in order to control populations for the purpose of maximizing security and wealth. The history of public health demonstrates its complicity both with the police and with capital.[4] It surveys the population in order to identify threats to the body politic, at the same time that it serves the need for a healthy labor force. The aim is not merely to control life, but to make it productive. The noble and essential role of the knowledges, technologies, and institutions of public health in reducing mortality from accidents, infectious disease, maternity, and in childhood gets entangled with poverty, race, and sexual difference. A metaphorics of contagion and contamination, of threat and death, authorizes racially marked and sexually differentiated policies of detention and discipline. Correction officers, correction facilities, and corrective treatments and surgeries ensure that the wayward are *led straight*. (*Correct:* fr. L *correctus,* pp. of *corrigere,* fr. *com-* + *regere* to lead straight.)

Global capital, both licit and illicit, grafts onto this normalizing apparatus infrastructures for the profitable harvesting of humanbodies. Rousseau would limit social inequity by the rule that no one should be so poor as to need to sell himself, nor so rich as to be able to buy another; nonetheless, if slavery has diminished and can no longer be defended, humanbodies have become increasingly capitalized.[5] Beyond the easy complicity of capital and public health around security and the productivity of labor, sex trafficking and prostitution are no longer cottage industries, but thriving global businesses. Women's bodies are used to sell everything from cars to dish soap. New medical technologies have given rise to markets in organs and genetic materials. New reproductive technologies have made it possible for women to sell their services as surrogates or egg sources. At a time of increasing social inequity, capitalization enjoys powerful new technical strategies and claims more and more bodies.

Relying on the discourse of rights, bioethics tends to address these issues in individual terms, as if the issue were the man's right to donate a kidney or a woman's right to choose to be a surrogate. An analysis of *biopower* reveals the way in which individual choice is always set within a culture of possibilities.[6] It exposes the infrastructures of life that determine what can be said, done, and thought and by whom, as well as the way in which social inequity determines opportunity. Individual liberty is not so much constrained by these infrastructures as constituted by them. As Adam established his dominion over the animals by naming them, so too those agencies that have the power to wield general names, the authority to provide theories of truth, or the right to govern life by delimiting specific identities control the diagnostic practices that assign actual human lives to those destinies: man, woman, savage, poor, mad.

The possibility of reimagining the infrastructures of life to promote a more livable and just future depends not only on a critique of the discourse of rights but also on an analysis of its complicity with biopower. Paying attention to the exclusions that establish the subject of rights and to the practices that enforce them, a critical phenomenology aims to undermine the hegemony of capital over life and to make the familiar strange by exposing the link between the forces that have turned the world into "one vast market" and the rights of Man.

FROM SOVEREIGN POWER TO BIOPOLITICS: CONCEPTUALIZATION, SEXUALIZATION, AND CAPITALIZATION

Foucault's historical analyses locate the difference between the "Classical" and the "Modern" ages at the end of the eighteenth century, when sovereign power gives way to biopower, governmentality, and biopolitics.[7] Sovereign power operated vertically to exercise the right of life and death. As Hobbes and Rousseau argued, if the sovereign commands that the citizen be put to death, the citizen should submit willingly, as he exists only in virtue of a social contract or covenant that creates sovereign power by investing it with the right "to take life or let live." Exercising the "right of the sword,"[8] sovereign power regulates the right to property through his power to dispose of a man and all his possessions.[9]

Modernity takes shape, as the singularity of sovereign power is at once absorbed and displaced by a multiplicity of institutions, agencies, codes, and policies with the right, not to take life or let live, but to "make live" or "let die." The undifferentiated hierarchical power of the sovereign to dispose of life descends via the naming and the commanding of the individual. Biopower disperses itself laterally across populations in microtechniques that manage the interface of words and bodies to secure safety and property. Instead of the right to take life, these new administrative agencies are charged with managing or controlling life in order to promote public health and maximize wealth. In place of the sovereign's judgment and fear of death, modern Man submits to surveillance and regulation according to public norms of security and productivity. While violence is regularized or subject to law under sovereign power, *life* is regularized under biopower.

Emphasizing the disjunction between the classical and modern ages, Foucault frequently suppresses the continuity of sovereign power with biopower. "Sovereign Power's effect on life is exercised only when the sovereign can kill."[10] This ignores the way in which prescriptions of sexual propriety are, from the very beginning, irretrievably intertwined with the right to property. Indeed, it is a symptom of a more general blindness on Foucault's part to the rhizomatous nature of the gender division of labor. Hobbes and Rousseau both insist that sovereign power enjoys not only the right to kill but also the right to decide what is proper to Man. Sexual difference and the gender division of labor permeate every aspect of life. The transition between the two periods is not so much a disjunct between two distinct forms of life, as Foucault himself admits,[11] but a radical transformation, like one of Dionysus' metamorphoses, produced by the dispersal of sovereign power, sometimes gradual and sometimes abrupt, into corporate agencies charged to regulate and control life.[12]

Disciplinary power mediates the metamorphosis of sovereign power into biopower. At the end of the eighteenth century, the singularity of sovereign power begins to be "govermentalized" or dispersed in a bureaucracy of state and nonstate agencies. Continuous with the hierarchical power of the sovereign "to take life or let live," there emerges a new "power of regularization" aimed at "making live and letting die."[13] Regularization grafts obedience to the law onto the techniques and procedures for making life productive.

Medicine holds a special place in Foucault's analysis as it provides the primary site of this transformation, the site where the individual is redefined as a member of a population. The possibility of the anatomico-pathological method and modern nosology arises when the sick are redistributed in a homogeneous physical and conceptual space where the regularities of the form of the disease can be discovered, as the physician finds it again and again across a field of cases. As the first "scientific discourse concerning the individual," medicine undermines the classical opposition between universal and particular by focusing on the judgment of the case.[14] Medical knowledge is not equivalent to the taxonomy of disease, nor to the principles of physiology; rather, clinical judgment is the scene of its deployment. The universal or form of disease must be known in its manifestation in this specific individual; otherwise, it is a mere abstraction. At the same time, the individual's legibility depends on considering him as a member of a population, a case of pleurisy or gout.

This "anatomo-politics" gives rise to various disciplinary technologies focused on the management of individual bodies. The surveillance and segregation of bodies in prisons, hospitals, and asylums secures the border between the normal and the pathological. The body politic exercises the right to invoke a *cordon sanitaire* to protect itself from the individual's diseased body. Public health depends on this alliance of police and physicians, on a partnership of agents of security and agents of medicine.[15] At the same time, a "disciplinary technology of labor" maximizes productivity through drilling, training, scheduling, and assessing individual workers. Disciplinary power reconceptualizes the individual as a member of a population, at the same time that its techniques remain focused on the individual body as a point of intervention.

What distinguishes biopower is intervention at the level not of the body but the species. The "anatomo-politics" of disciplinary power is replaced by a "'biopolitics' of the human race."[16] Disciplinary power "tries to rule a multiplicity of men to the extent that their multiplicity can and must be dissolved into individual bodies that can be kept under surveillance, trained, used, and if need be, punished," while biopower "is addressed to a multiplicity of men, not to the extent that they are nothing more than their individual bodies, but to the extent that they form, on the contrary, a global mass that is affected by overall processes characteristic of birth, death, production, illness, and so on."[17] Biopower completes the progressive abstraction initiated by the discourse of rights and the articulation of abstract names. Disciplinary power knows the individual as a member of a population while treating him as a distinct body. Biopower develops techniques and strategies for the disposal of whole populations.[18] In the regulation of production and reproduction, it is characterized not so much by prescriptions for normalizing individuals, though disciplinary power remains its key technique, as by policies and agencies aimed at the assignment and management of life as a military and economic resource.

Biopower subordinates the disciplinary concern with normalcy and pathology to the values of security and economic productivity. Under biopower, life is "governmentalized." It is subject to surveillance, bookkeeping, and management not only by the governmentalized state and its policies but also by powerful nonstate actors as well, such as civic or professional associations, business entities, or transnational agencies. Governmentalization depends on the development of "apparatuses" for the administration of security and productivity informed by the expert knowledges (savoirs) required to manage populations.[19]

Biopolitics emerges with political economy at the nexus of politics, law, and economics where human life will be reinterpreted both as commodified labor and as human capital.[20] It rests on "two great ensembles of political knowledge and technology": on the one hand, the concepts, techniques, and strategies of diplomacy and the military; on the other, those like economics, statistics, and medicine that aim to increase wealth and productivity.[21] "Commerce and monetary circulation" operate at the "junction point" of these military and economic apparatuses. Biopolitics aims to exploit the connection between population and wealth. Governmentality, the deployment of biopower to serve the aims of biopolitics, attempts to maximize the population and protect its health to ensure adequately large military forces and an adequate supply of healthy, able workers. Agencies and policies regulate nutrition, urban planning, housing, sanitation, and family planning, monitor birthrates and unemployment, and identify and target those subpopulations that can be "let die," the civilian casualties in military operations, for example, or the chronically poor who are not economically productive.

The conceptualization of the individual as a member of a population enables the disposition, all at once, of a class of bodies. This way of thinking, so necessary to scientific medicine, when transposed into politics replaces the actual individual with an abstraction for the purpose of facilitating his disposition in accord with security and productivity. Reducing a human life to a unit in a calculus of military and economic probabilities contradicts the idea of a bioethics, an ethics of life. An ethics that subordinates life to violence and property is no bioethics.

This conceptualization, which reduces the individual to a case, goes hand in hand with a thoroughgoing sexualization of experience. "Population-wealth" is the "privileged object of the new governmental reason."[22] Commerce and monetary circulation make possible an increase in population, which, in turn, increases "manpower, production, and export, and [the possibility] of endowing oneself with large, powerful armies."[23] The governmentalized state has an interest in managing the intimacies of reproduction to maximize labor and human capital. Public health advances not only through its policing function but also through "campaigns" aimed at intervening in sexual practices and family planning in order to manage birthrates and child rearing.[24] In the nineteenth century, the "disease" of masturbation became an urgent focus of medicine and public health, as it supposedly sapped vitality and endangered productivity and capital.

By the 1830s, infantile sexuality was already accorded an "inexhaustible causal power."[25] Everything from infertility to insanity could be traced to masturbation. Masturbation, the "total illness," acts as an etiology across the nosological categories. It can affect fertility, the digestive functions, the heart, the nervous system, and rate of growth, as well as attitude and character. It makes a man "fickle and capricious," "feeble," and "unable to fix his attention on any subject, or to pursue any active employment," if not infertile and insane. It can lead him to attempt castration.[26] Masturbation provided a ubiquitous causality that "enables everything that is otherwise inexplicable to be explained."[27] Even a man's old age and death may be attributed to a "premature exhaustion of his organism" caused by masturbation.[28] The effects of masturbation extend across the whole of Man's life. Indeed, many physicians shared the view of M. Réveillé-Parise: "In my opinion, neither the plague, nor war, nor smallpox, nor a crowd of similar evils, have resulted more disastrously for humanity, than the habit of masturbation: it is the destroying element of civilized society."[29] Sexuality exerts its causality not only over the whole being of the person but over culture and history itself.

The stage is set for psychoanalysis and its consolidation of the sexualization of experience, culture, and history. Psychoanalysis insists not only on the analogy between "the processes of civilization and the libidinal development of the individual" but also on a thorough sexualization of the relation of mother and child.[30] The mother is the infant's first "*love*-object," a love marked by the "repression" of "a part of his [*sic*] sexual aims."[31] Though Freud is careful to distinguish infantile sexuality from genital sexuality, the two are continuous. In his account the latter is already implicit in the former. Female sexuality and the mother-daughter relation remain unthought and invisible in this hypothetical story.[32]

The urgent concern about infantile sexuality and masturbation emerges at the same time that the heterosexual family is installed through institutions and policies as the basic social unit. "At the very moment that the cellular family is enclosed in a dense, affective space, it is endowed with a rationality that, in the name of illness, plugs it into a technology, into an external medical power and knowledge. The new substantial, affective, and sexual family is at the same time a medicalized family."[33] At the end of the eighteenth century, the family had become an object of study for medicine, education, the social sciences, and state policy. Experts and expert knowledge are required to establish the "schema of rationality" that will ensure the "survival . . . training and normalized development" of the family's children. "In short, a series of technical authorities supervise and dominate the family itself."[34] Ironically, while mothers require the tutelage of the experts and their expert knowledge, they are nevertheless accountable for their children's condition and obliged to ameliorate it. Mothers are enjoined to spy on their children and to form a "single body" with them, "an urgent folding of the [mothers'] bodies over their children's bodies."[35] At the same time, any discovery must be immediately handed over to the experts.[36] Just as Rousseau held a wife absolutely responsible for her husband's happiness while denying her any agency of her own, so too the new science of sexuality holds the mother absolutely responsible without according her any authority whatsoever.

Surveillance provides the first line of defense against masturbation. A chronic masturbator suffers as he does due to the inattention and failure of vigilance on the part of his caregiver.[37] If the mother or the nurse, her substitute, had kept the child properly under surveillance, he would not have had the opportunity to develop the habit. The family is reconfigured as a "space of surveillance," and parental care consists in deploying a variety of strategies by which to catch the child in the act.[38] Foucault repeats the story of a boy who is put to bed with bells on so that, should he begin to masturbate, he would wake his older brother who could then prevent him from touching himself.[39] The new science of sexuality places the relation between mother and child under a constant threat and transforms care into a form of monitoring on behalf of the experts and on behalf of the state's interest in the child's productivity. The state puts the family under surveillance by subverting mothering and generativity into a principle and agency of surveillance, diagnosis, and disposition, while it redirects the aims of the family toward population wealth.[40]

If surveillance fails, more drastic measures must be applied. For boys, these included a variety of mostly reversible measures. Börner favored the regulation of diet and the avoidance of anything "hot or heat-producing."[41] Vogel recommended more drastic measures to prevent the boy from touching himself, including locking underwear or a restraining harness.[42] Foucault notes the use of splints and even the insertion of tubes or needles in the boy's penis to make masturbation impossible.[43] It became a common practice for doctors to appear before a particularly recalcitrant case with a pair of large scissors threatening to cut off his genitals.[44]

For women who were deemed intransigent cases, the removal of genitalia was no mere threat, but the contemporary physician's idea of best practice. When the doctor brandished his knife, it was no pantomime. Deslandes, the author of *De l'onanisme,* likens clitoredectomy to "amputating the infected limb to save the whole."[45] He argues that the removal of the clitoris constitutes no "disadvantage" to a woman, insofar as she likely belongs to "'the already very large category' of women who are 'insensitive' to the pleasures of love." This "insensitivity," he notes, is not incompatible with a faithful execution of their marital and maternal duties. The last documented clitoredectomy in the United States was performed in 1948 on a five year old as a cure for masturbation.[46]

Medical theories of the nineteenth century both in Europe and the United States ascribed a pancausality to the ovaries and female reproductive organs. Both a woman's psychology and her physiology were understood to be at the mercy of them.[47] Physicians consistently described women as teetering on the edge of insanity, hysteria, and even crime due to "her body's peculiar dominance."[48]

Women of relative means and liberty, who might have engaged in intellectual endeavors, were proscribed from doing so. Thinking, like masturbation, would sap the energy needed for reproduction. As the German neurologist Paul Moebius warned, "If we wish woman to fulfill the task of motherhood fully she cannot possess a masculine brain ... her material organs would suffer and we should have before us a repulsive and useless hybrid."[49] In the United States during the second half of the nineteenth century, women who failed to be led straight into this identity were often diagnosed with "female invalidism" and subjected to a range of treatments from extended bed rest and isolation to surgical interventions.[50] In her short story about her own experience of the "rest cure," Charlotte Perkins Gilman repeatedly remarks that if she were only allowed to work, to write down her thoughts, she would feel much better, but, to her family and physicians, that activity is both the symptom and the cause of her illness.[51]

Physicians argued against higher education, suffrage, and intellectual activity for women not only because these activities would undermine her reproductive capacities but also because they were intrinsically "unwomanly," inconsistent with a woman's nature. These activities would disturb her delicate equilibrium, her fragile perch on the edge between nature and culture, perhaps tipping her into hysteria or insanity.[52] Though medical theory ascribed to women little or no sexual appetite, her sexuality determines who she can be and explains her existence throughout. If physicians thought masturbation to be less frequent among girls than boys, when a girl was discovered to be a masturbator, it was a much greater calamity as it threatened both her nature and her value in the marriage market. The surveillance that marriageable girls have always been under must be extended over little girls as well. Masturbation might threaten a boy's health, but the autoeroticism of masturbation threatened a girl's very identity, both by contradicting her natural modesty and asexuality and by directing her sexuality toward herself and her own pleasure, rather than preserving it for her husband. The sexualization of experience in the nineteenth century reinforced women's status as property. Women's sexuality was already subject to the laws of the market.

Capital and capitalism, Foucault argues, depend upon biopower. Capitalism "would not have been possible without the controlled insertion of bodies into the machinery of production and the adjustment of the phenomena of population to economic processes."[53] Biopower provides the material infrastructures of capital by disposing of bodies in order to maximize security and the accumulation of wealth. The anatomo- and biopolitics that emerged in the last half of the eighteenth century comprised "techniques of power" that intervene "at every level of the social body" and regulate "very diverse institutions," including not only the family but also the army, schools, police, public health, medicine, and other collective and governmental agencies. All these formations, however, served "economic processes, their development, and the forces working to sustain them."[54] As "factors of segregation and social hierarchization," these techniques produced "relations of domination and effects of hegemony." Alongside the still vital relations of mastery and slavery, there emerges a diffuse, invasive, laterally dispersed power aimed at the maximization of populations and productivity. Biopower "join[s] the growth of human groups to the expansion of productive forces and the differential allocation of profit."[55] It creates new identities to regulate the behavior of populations in line with the aims of capital: worker, student, patient, consumer. To maximize population wealth, the "accumulation of men" must be adjusted to the "accumulation of capital." Women must be prevented from engaging in intellectual activity, because their reproductive capacities are essential to capital and must be maximized and, to that end, regularized by science and law. If, as Foucault argues, with the emergence of biopower "the life of the species is wagered on its own political strategies," then it is with the body of a woman that the bet is made.

THE CAPITALIZATION OF LIFE

The difference between the sexes, to anyone who cares to examine this human dimension with a little objectivity, has been reduced to a question of money, like everything else.

—LUCE IRIGARAY, "A CHANCE TO LIVE" (1989)

Since Eve, the female body has been a disrupting influence on men. Provoking his appetite, a woman's body undermines the detachment, power of abstraction, and self-reliance that define the Man of reason.

Historically, this danger has been addressed with a combination of spatial confinement and dress codes. The mobility of a woman in Saudi Arabia is carefully regulated, and she must be invisible in the public space, unseen except by her husband or male guardian and those he permits. This immobility and invisibility preclude real citizenship or participation in public activities and the councils that determine the future, so that the dress code reinforces a woman's status as property, while undermining her agency.

Similarly, anxiety about the effect of girls' bodies on boys has spawned a wave of dress codes in U.S. middle schools. Typically, middle school includes the sixth to eighth grades, children from eleven to thirteen years of age or preteens. Many U.S. middle schools enforce the "fingertip rule": with her arms at her sides, a girl's shorts must extend at least to her fingertips. The strictness and consistency with which the rule is enforced depends on the school, but failure to pass the test can provoke discipline. In 2012 a sixth grader at Maplewood Middle School in New Jersey who failed the test was "pulled from class and sent to detention, where she was ordered to don a Hester Prynne–style 'shirt of shame' for the rest of the school day—an oversized men's shirt that covered her from neck to shins."[56] Ironically, the girl had asked her mother to take a picture of her earlier in the day because she had a solo in a school concert that evening and wanted to commemorate the day. Her mother cites her "enthusiasm" and "confidence" at the time of the photo and argues that such disciplinary policies are undermining that confidence and teaching girls to be ashamed of themselves and their bodies. She reports a "barrage" of communications in the school district regarding dress codes that specifically identify the problem as particular to female students. School officials justify the dress code policies by alluding to the degree to which the girls' dress is disrupting the "learning environment." At Morris Knolls High School in New Jersey, where the students are fifteen to eighteen years of age, the students protested the local dress code policy, arguing that it promotes a "rape culture:" "Our dress code bans 'suggestive clothing,' which perpetuates the myth that women are raped because of what they wear, that exposing their skin means they are 'asking for it'. . . . It also suggests male students cannot be held responsible for their behavior if presented with such 'distracting' clothing. This is rape culture. Why does the administration support it?"[57]

On July 12, 2014, the front page of the *New York Times* presented two cases of rape. In the right-hand column ran a news story about a young girl in India who had been raped by the male relatives of a woman of higher caste. Apparently, the woman had been harassed by the girl's brother. Her rape was ordered by tribal elders to settle the dispute. It took place very publicly with the awareness of her village.

Boxed in the center of the front page ran a feature story about a rape that had taken place on a college campus months earlier. At first, the rape of the college freshman appears quite different from the rape of the Indian villager. The latter was blameless. The college student had been drinking and was significantly impaired by alcohol. Though the men involved initially made false statements, ultimately there was no dispute that various sex acts had taken place involving the freshman girl and several members of the football team. The college must have believed that the young woman's involvement was consensual, as the men who engaged sexually with her were exonerated by the college's review process. Despite her incapacitation and the evidence of rough sex, the college judged that the woman had not been assaulted.

The two cases might appear morally distinct, but both incidents reflect a pervasive "rape culture," the ubiquitous disposability of the female body under the narrative of the social contract and rights of Man. In both cases the very communal structures that are supposed to ensure justice for the vulnerable are complicit in the violence that is done to these victims. These agencies reinforce the female body's position at the disposal of men. Perhaps it is the object of a man's lascivious gaze, like Emile's governor, who undresses in his imagination the modestly attired young girl. Perhaps it is a terrible source of temptation that must be covered up because it provokes men to lust and violence. Perhaps it is a generative and nourishing space to be fenced off and possessed like a piece of land, an ownership marked by the fact that Man gives his name to both, designating something not to be violated by the other men / brothers. Perhaps it is a profit center of labor and consumption. The girls of Morris Knolls High have exposed the strategic complicity of the dress codes and "rape culture" in managing the value and threat of the female body.

The high school dress codes expose the specific difference of biopower. If the female body has always been a contested site, the sexualization of experience grafts onto the apparatus of the rights of man and the law of property the idea of managing the female body to enhance productivity, at the same time that it increases its vulnerability to violence. In the rationale of the dress codes, girls' bodies constantly threaten to disturb boys' productivity. Female bodies, *as a population*, must be managed to diffuse the danger. Moreover, if the girls' bodies have a negative relation to productivity from which it must be protected, they also have a positive relation to productivity as profit centers. The medicalization of sexuality and the reduction of a woman to her reproductive organs serve the governmental interest in population wealth. Woman remains a threat, but that threatening sexuality can be put to work: tamed and made productive.

The girls reflect these apparently contradictory forces. They want to wear the midriff tops and short shorts because *it is the fashion* for women to display their sexuality.[58] *Teen Vogue*'s "Top 12 Fall Fashion Trends" includes very short skirts, short shorts, midriff tops, very tight jeans, as well as very tight and torn jeans.[59] Multibillion-dollar industries depend on and cultivate the teen and preteen markets.[60] Investment banks and asset management firms identify the teen clothing business as a growing and lucrative market. Analysts estimate that American teenagers spend an average of four thousand dollars annually, over 30 percent of it on clothing, their largest budget category. The girls' sexuality, like everything else in our culture, is subject to the "unconditional power of money."[61]

Criticism in the media of this economic formation of children tends to focus not on the marketing strategies that create the demand, nor on industry profits, nor on the way in which this sexualization of young girls may affect their "confidence" and "enthusiasm." Rather, the reporting reflects the culture's own anxiety about female sexuality. On the one hand, it makes some people "uncomfortable"; on the other it puts the girl herself at risk, either of provoking male aggression or of being disciplined for creating a disturbance.[62] While this market profits from the girls, the old rules remain in place, and a girl's modesty must be carefully regulated to balance productivity and security. In the complicity of sexualization and capitalization, a girl's own "confidence" and "enthusiasm" figure as elements of a marketing plan, rather than as commanding values. Enough sex to make a profit, but not so much as to unleash the disruptive force: no doubt the manipulation of a girl's "confidence" and "enthusiasm" proves a useful strategy in regulating this productive balance. As Baudrillard argues, production under capitalization is "never just the production of goods; it is always also the production of relations and of differences. . . . A deep logical collusion links the mega-corporation and the micro-consumer."[63] Advertising capitalizes on the ideology of individuality to produce and reproduce customers who will conform to the code of consumption, including the young girls of Maplewood, New Jersey.

The market research firm IbisWorld estimates that the women's clothing market in the United States produces 44 billion dollars in revenue annually, supporting 30,000 businesses and employing more than 360 thousand workers.[64] This market exhibits the same chiasm of sexualization and discipline around women's bodies as the children's market. While women in Saudi Arabia are rendered invisible by their dress codes, limitations on women's mobility and agency in Anglo-European countries are associated with an overexposure of the female body. The promiscuous circulation throughout these cultures of images that hypersexualize and subjugate the female body—such as the Calvin Klein advertisement featuring the actress Eva Mendes in a position of subjection suggesting bondage[65]—works to delegitimate the participation of women in the discursive domains of science, politics, and philosophy, as well as in the practical counsels of politicians, financiers, and opinionators where the future is determined. This is not the image of a world leader. This disciplined and overexposed female body serves the same aims as the Saudi dress codes for women, though via different microtechniques of biopower. Such an image does not promote the mobility and agency of women, rather it reinscribes woman as disciplined sexuality to maximize profit.

If Saudi dress codes are linked to a lack of mobility and agency, so are Western fashions. In 2009 the runways of international haute couture fashion shows were littered with models who fell trying to walk in shoes that were not made to sustain mobility. On *New York Magazine*'s fashion blog *The Cut*, Amy Odell commented that,

judging by the spring 2009 shoes we've seen on the runway so far, one might think designers had it in for us ladies. Because these heels are so high they're scary. Nay—*dangerous.* They've alrady caused models to fall at Rodarte, Prada, and Pucci. And still more models reported stumbling at Dolce & Gabanna,

BCBG, and Peter Som. Models survived the Basso & Brooke, Marni, and Christian Dior shows unscathed, but that doesn't mean the cat walkers weren't scared walking in them. Next spring's hottest accessory may just be a pair of crutches.[66]

As Bill Cunningham remarks in the *New York Times* Style section, "Designers can upset the whole world. But today it's the shoe designers who turn things upside down."[67] Cunningham observes several women trying to walk in platform shoes without heels, including the beer heiress Daphne Guinness. Guinness leaned against a building "so as not to fall over," while she waited for her car and chauffeur, who had to help her to the car, as *she could not walk on her own.*[68]

Dozens of pictures of models falling can be found on the internet. Particularly interesting is a scene from the Fall 2009 Hervé Léger show. It included numerous falls by models attempting to walk in shoes that did not sustain mobility, but one photo captures the capitalization of the model's body in the indifference of every spectator to her plight and her injury.[69] As she falls and is caught on the camera at the level of the feet of those sitting in the front row, not a toe twitches. No one moves to aid her or shows any concern, though apparently the audience did clap when the models recovered and moved down the runway.[70] When asked about the falls, the designer Max Azria remarked, "I don't care. If people talk about that instead of the clothes, that would be ridiculous."[71] Azria's style is known as "sex on heels," and he is also the designer who makes "second-skin dresses that make it hard to sit down."[72]

International haute couture fashion models may not be the most sympathetic constituency for an analysis of labor injustice, but the capitalization of these women's bodies exhibits the role of microtechniques like fashion in constricting the agency and mobility of women and in installing and enforcing their exclusion from the public processes determining our collective future. These models do not so much sell their labor as yield their very bodies to the production process and to the often cruel pleasure of the spectator, much as surrogate mothers marketed in various medical tourism industries yield themselves to the surveillance and regulation of for-profit clinics. The models are subject to a constant microsurveillance of the body. They work long hours for low pay without benefits or any regulation in the workplace. They are subject to erratic schedules, arduous travel, and high injury rates, as well as unhealthy practices related to maintaining abnormally low weights. They are frequently victims of sexual abuse. Racism and other prejudices determine hiring. They are subject to degrading and demeaning situations on and off the runway. If unsympathetic, these models nonetheless provide a surprisingly acute example of the sexualized capitalization of the female body and its relation to women's disenfranchisement in the public sphere.[73] Bioethics, an ethics of life, surely ought to concern itself with this conjunction of health, labor, and injustice; yet, by focusing narrowly on issues raised by "progress in science," bioethics makes no place for these women's lives in its agenda.

More interest has been shown to medical tourism, transnational reproductive travel, and the growing transnational surrogacy industry. Though commentators repeatedly cite the lack of good data, medical tourism is estimated to be worth 60 billion dollars annually.[74] In India alone—the largest market for transnational surrogacy—the industry is thought to produce revenues between 500 million and 2.3 billion dollars. This is no accident, but the effect of a self-conscious business deal between the state and medicine to produce foreign capital. In his 2003–2004 budget, Jaswant Singh, India's Minister of Finance and Company Affairs, presented a long-term development program for positioning India as a "global health destination."[75] In the last ten years medical tourism has realized Singh's aim, proving to be one of India's most important sources of economic growth and foreign capital.

In place of India's traditional public health care system, the economic success of this alliance has produced two systems, a private one for international clients or wealthy Indians and a series of public "health missions" for the poor and rural populations. India's first for-profit hospital opened in 2005, marketing "First World Health-Care at Emerging Market Prices."[76] The success of Singh's development program has exacerbated already extreme health and social inequities.

> The past decade has seen growing inequalities in access to health care. On the one hand, corporate hospitals with state-of-the-art facilities cater to the elite and attract foreign patients, creating medical tourism as a new economic entity that gets undue policy attention in the National Health Policy 2002. On the other hand, the majority are left to market forces, and medical expenditure is the second highest cause of rural indebtedness. Health indicators like the infant mortality rate have stagnated or even worsened in some large states, despite growing national wealth.[77]

This is the context in which Indian women are marketed as surrogate mothers to a largely Anglo-European clientele.

Though the Indian Council of Medical Research has issued guidelines for the surrogacy market, the clinics are largely unregulated.[78] Procedures for obtaining consent are not standardized. The women recuited by the for-profit clinics are mostly extremely poor and illiterate, and consent may be compromised by poor understanding. Payment schemes are not standardized, and surrogates may be made to "shoulder the risk of producing a suboptimal product."[79] Clients pay fifteen to twenty thousand dollars, while the surrogate receives usually about six thousand dollars, but lower payments are not uncommon. Clinics may or may not pay the money directly to the women themselves, who may or may not be able to retain control of the money if it is paid to them and who may or may not have the resources to manage it if they do.

What protocols do exist actively isolate the surrogate from clients as well as from donors if the surrogate is not also supplying the egg. A surrogate is immediately separated from the child at birth to minimize any attachment. They are regularly isolated in hostels attached to the for-profit clinics, where they are put under surveillance and subjected to various regimens of diet, exercise, and medical assessment.

These techniques of isolation, surveillance, and discipline form an important part of the marketing campaigns of the clinics. An American client expressed the sales appeal: "[In the United States] you have no idea if your surrogate mother is smoking, drinking alcohol, doing drugs. You don't know what she's doing. You have a third-party agency as a mediator between the two of you, but *there's no one policing her.*"[80] The surrogate's body is both a site of productivity and a security risk.

Some feminist commentators have argued that criticisms of the Indian surrogacy industry amount to paternalism, if not imperialism. Certainly, as Alison Jaggar has argued, the condition of women in the developing world reflects, in large part, the forces of global capital rather than their own culture.[81] The coalition of private health care providers and the Indian government has pursued this growth strategy only because surrogacy is a lucrative market driven by the demand for biological reproduction in Anglo-European countries and other wealthy populations.[82] For this very reason, the policy calls for philosophical critique: state policy recruits poor and vulnerable women into an apparatus that degrades local health care and transforms their bodies into sites for the production of foreign capital. The client may obtain a baby, but the real advantage goes to the apparatus itself and the accumulation of power and wealth for the private / public partnership.

There is nothing intrinsically wrong with surrogacy motherhood: a friend or relative might offer to serve as a surrogate out of altruism without any ethical harm or injustice being done.[83] As Ruth Macklin has argued, the "moral flaws are tied to the commercial features of surrogacy, not the arrangement itself."[84] Macklin rightly insists that the assessment of reproductive tourism in India ought to be based on "factual circumstances," including the quality of care the surrogate receives during and after the pregnancy as well as the fairness of her compensation and the reliability that it will be paid. More recently, Macklin has found the claim that surrogates in India are exploited unconvincing, insofar as surrogacy provides a lucrative option for individual women who are extremely poor and have few opportunities.[85] Such payments, Macklin argues, are not "coercive," as the surrogates are offered a "desirable option" rather than two negative options: "Your money or your life!" In fact, the surrogate is presented with similarly undesirable options: sell us your life, your generativity, or you will remain crushingly poor.[86] No one "desires" to be a surrogate, as surrogacy is not in itself desirable. The "desirable option" would be to have the opportunity to achieve economic independence through sustainable work without the need to put her generativity at the service of the state and global capital.

The government has introduced an incentive that is out of proportion in a world of few or no options and thus inevitably compelling, if not coercive. Moreover, the aim of this state policy is not to benefit the surrogates but to profit the public / private partnership. The surrogate is exploited not because she is threatened, nor because she is paid too much or too little, nor because she receives less than her share of advantage from the relationship, but because she belongs to a system of exploitation that treats her generativity as a cost of production. The surrogate will receive a level and quality of care in the pregnancy that she would have no hope of receiving in a pregnancy of her own. Her state has invested in technology and expertise to which she will have access only in order to benefit the client and produce profit for the public / private partnership. Justice requires the state to treat her generativity, not as a resource, but as its aim: what would be required for this woman to give birth in security and against the horizon of a sustainable future for herself and her child? How would the infrastructures of generativity be configured differently and how would the relation of individual women to citizenship and the state be transformed if the state and the public / private partnership had invested these resources in maternal / child health and the education of girls?

The population wealth apparatus intervenes in individual lives not to improve them but to make them productive for capital. The surrogate is exploited because the state makes policy that does not address her needs, while relying on her as a material condition of production. Both the state and the client exploit her poverty. Surrogacy in India costs 20 percent less than in the United States, and this is what drives the transnational market.[87] The clients *take advantage* of the low cost, and the public / private partnership *takes advantage* of the high profit, and both advantages derive from the surrogates' poverty and vulnerability.

The argument that the surrogate is nonetheless benefited by the arrangement ignores the fact that surrogacy neither provides nor leads to sustainable work. The surrogate does not learn skills or acquire knowledge or participate in experiences that will enable her to attain an economically independent future. In return for work that reinforces her status as sexualized property, she receives a one-time payment that may be adequate to buy a house or send her son to school, but she will still be poor and without the resources to address that poverty.

The claim that the surrogate *chooses* to become a surrogate is as thin as her real options. Even if it were the case that the surrogate understood clearly the proposal, was not unduly targeted by the recruiters, and was not pressured by other parties, the extreme social inequity between the clients and clinics, on the one hand, and the surrogates, on the other, imply real choices and possibilities for the former and a bleakly limited future for the latter. Beyond the life of poverty all around her, surrogacy may seem like the *only* choice, which is to say no *choice* at all. The question of choice is not psychological, but structural. Freedom depends upon a *culture of possibilities*: institutions, practices, and relationships that support the flourishing of each and all. "That in the name of individual rights someone is allowed to do as he wants, great! But if what we want to do is to create a new way of life [*mode de vie*] then the question of individual rights is not pertinent."[88] Focusing only on the individual surrogate and defending her "right to choose" to be a surrogate without analyzing the poverty and disempowerment that condition this "choice" hardly does her justice, nor does it create a "new way of life" for her.

Macklin also rightly criticizes arguments against India's surrogacy industry that rely on the idea of commodification. As she points out, the commodification of the body is not specific to gestational surrogacy.[89] Almost all humans are obliged to sell their time as labor. The surrogates' bodies, however, are not only commodified but also capitalized. Their very bodies become profit centers, just as do those of fashion models. What distinguishes the surrogates, however, is the capitalization of their generativity, that element of existence by which each woman is joined to the universal. "I belong to the universal in recognizing that I am a woman . . . Belonging to a gender represents a universal that exists prior to me."[90] The distinct generativity of her gender distinguishes a woman from a man, so that "human nature is [at least] two." Through the solidarity of her gender, a woman participates in her generativity as something universal.

Women share with men the plasticity of the brain, hand, and foot, and the difference from other animals that destiny is not prefigured in the *differentiae*, but they are distinguished from men, and yet bound to one another, by their generativity. All women are comprised by the possibility of pregnancy, whether that possibility is thwarted by infertility or spectacular, as in the case of transwomen who, appearing as women, might very well appear as someone's mother. The biology of the female sex reminds women early on and frequently of their capacity for pregnancy. These reminders require sufficient attention that whole industries thrive around them. In some cultures, women have been required to isolate themselves during menstruation to manage the threat of their sexuality and its polluting power. Girls know, early on, that these reminders also signal their vulnerability to sexual aggression and unwanted pregnancy. Beyond the war of all against all and the right to property, a phenomenology of this generativity provides a new universal starting point for ethics.

Under the rights of Man and social contract theory, the distinctive generativity of female humans is appropriated by men in the rhetoric of "conception" and the fiction of nature as Man's Mother. At the same time, women's actual labor remains undervalued and unrecognized. Women are both defined by and as their reproductive capacity, while that power is rendered something utterly particular, without any implications for ethics or politics. Women are nothing but reproduction, but that activity offers no figures of the universally human.

Under the thought of sexual difference, the inverse is true. Her generativity is only an element of a woman's existence, not continuous with it, while that generativity is, at the same time, something universal or human. With the recognition of the irreducibility of sexual difference comes the impossibility of thinking the universal under the logic of the one or the generic. The universal will be at least two, and more. The visibility of women's generativity, on which the vitality of the community depends, makes possible new figures of ethical and political relationship. The evidence of women's experience and history, her generativity and reproductive labor, offer the opportunity to discover unheard of possibilities beyond property and sexual propriety.

In Anglo-European culture, the relationship of mother and child has almost always been figured as a relation of mother and son and articulated from the son toward the mother as *his* "love-object," passing over *her* generativity. The relation of mother and daughter figures this intergenerational generativity as a reciprocal "letting go" and "becoming like." The mother will let her daughter go to become a mother like herself. The purpose of mothering is to cultivate the other so that she may go free to become a generative force in her own right. A mother "folds her body over the other." She can bear another life inside herself in order to bring it to its own viability. Her love cultivates the other in every register of experience.[91] Her generativity is distinct from care labor. Though the concept of care labor has a universal significance in that everyone requires care during life, it has been developed largely in relation to disability and long-term care. Maternal generativity sustains the other with the explicit purpose of rendering that sustenance unnecessary. The freedom of the other is the end and aim. How would ethics and politics be refigured beginning from the universality of this intergenerational generativity?

CRITICAL PHENOMENOLOGY OF LIFE AS A PRACTICE OF FREEDOM

Social justice, and especially sexual justice, cannot be achieved without changing the laws of language and the conceptions of truths and values structuring the

social order. Changing the instruments of culture is just as important in the medium to long term as a redistribution of goods in the strict sense. You can't have one without the other.
—LUCE IRIGARAY, "HOW TO MANAGE THE TRANSITION
FROM NATURAL TO CIVIL COEXISTENCE?" (2001)

The critical ontology of ourselves must be considered not, certainly, as a theory, a doctrine, nor even as a permanent body of knowledge that is accumulating; it must be conceived as an attitude, an ethos, a philosophical life in which the critique of what we are is at one and the same time the historical analysis of the limits imposed on us and an experiment with the possibility of going beyond them [*de leur franchissement possible*]. . . . This task requires work on our limits, that is, a patient labor giving form to our impatience for liberty.
—MICHEL FOUCAULT, "WHAT IS ENLIGHTENMENT?" (1984)

Money should be spent trying out concepts that shatter our current structures and systems that have turned much of the world into one vast market. Is progress really Wi-Fi on every corner? No. It's when no 13-year-old girl on the planet gets sold for sex. But as long as most folks pat themselves on the back for charitable acts, we've got a perpetual poverty machine.
—PETER BUFFETT, "THE CHARITABLE-INDUSTRIAL COMPLEX" (2013)

Critical phenomenology takes up the "critique of what we are" as an "historical analysis of the limits imposed on us," but the "experiment with the possibility of going beyond them" requires that the critique be joined to the thought of the irreducibility of sexual difference. The critique focuses on the dependency of property and the rights of Man on the infrastructures of sexual propriety and the gender division of labor, as well as on the logic of abstraction that both installs Man as the figure of the generic and provides the general names by which Man disposes of women and other dependent or excluded populations. This "work carried out by ourselves upon ourselves as free beings" makes the familiar strange by exposing the contingent conditions that "led us to constitute ourselves and to recognize ourselves as subjects of what we are doing, thinking, saying."[92] The familiar invisibility of women in the collaborations and councils that determine the future and the familiar disposition of women's generativity in property and the gender division of labor must become strange in order to open up the possibility of going beyond them toward universals that promote this generativity for each and all.

Hobbes' philosopher engages in a "seeking" aimed at mastering nature, satisfying his appetites, and managing threat. An altogether different "curiosity" animates critical phenomenology. Curiosity combines "care for what exists" with "a certain determination to throw off familiar ways of thought and to look at the same things in a different way, a passion for seizing what is happening now and what is disappearing, a lack of respect for the traditional hierarchies of what is important and fundamental."[93]

The classical phenomenologist proposes a conceptual *epoché*, thinking the "suspension of the natural attitude" in order to arrive at the universal forms of a possible experience. The critical phenomenologist undertakes a material and conceptual *epoché*, paying attention to the specificity of the "natural attitude," the identities it prescribes and sustains, in order to discover new universals that respond to the urgencies of our time with new modes of life.[94] The critical phenomenologist analyses the images, metaphors, narratives, and theories in which identities are constituted and rights established as a way of tending and attending to life. The exposure of the apparatus that subordinates life to security and wealth aims at solidarity with all those agencies, activities, and practices that would invert the relationship.

Foucault contrasts his style of criticism with "passing judgment." Judgment disposes of a work or a life, assigning it to its proper place in a hierarchy from some privileged position of sovereignty. It assigns value or blame so as to settle accounts. Instead, Foucault imagines a nonsovereign criticism that would "bring an oeuvre, a book, a sentence, an idea to life."[95] Critical phenomenology is *of* life, not in that it represents life, but in that it works for life. It submits itself to life and promotes it.

Critique requires an unfamiliar attentiveness to life and its elements. It stills itself to "listen to the wind."[96] Air creates solidarity as a condition of life. Everyone breathes, but it takes stillness to hear it. Every mode of life has its air: the sharp mentholated scent of pine, the briny ocean breeze, the heavy sweetness of the bayou, or the clean aridity of the desert. Globalization and global capital threaten to eradicate this diversity of place and replace it with the homogeneity of toxic, unbreatheable air.

Critique "watches the grass grow." Nothing teaches patience like farming or gardening. The attempt to speed things up and make things bigger, faster, and more profitable more quickly threatens the vitality of the earth on which all life depends. Being *of* life, or on the side of life, requires a quiet attention to what exists and the patience to attend to life—to what comes into being, grows, and dies—as it displays itself in its own times and ways.

Critical phenomenology tries to "catch the sea foam in the breeze and scatter it." Water embodies the mobility of life and agency. Water runs, swirls, cascades, roils, boils, trickles, dribbles, splashes, pours. It pounds like an ocean wave or laps gently at the shoreline of a lake. It bubbles like a spring, flows like a river, and shoots and careens like a mountain creek. In some places, from time to time, it swamps or floods the earth or infuses the air with mist or thickens it with falling snow. Damming and commodifying water threaten its mobility and vitality, while destroying places and displacing peoples and other animals. The vitality of life depends on the integrity and mobility of water.

Critique "lights fires." Critical phenomenology ignites the metamorphic powers of life to make the familiar strange and to disturb the functioning of the population-wealth apparatus. It kindles not judgments but "signs of existence," marks of life, "[dragging] them from their sleep."[97] Classical phenomenology speculates timeless "formal structures" or the "universal conditions of [all] knowledge or all possible moral action" or a "metaphysics that has finally become a science." Critical phenomenology stokes the fiery signs of life in the apparatus, those moments where life escapes its management by biopower and its service to security and wealth, like the girls of Morris Knolls High.

By exposing the contingency of the familiar, criticism awakens "the possibility of being otherwise: it will separate out, from the contingency that has made us what we are, the possibility of no longer being, doing, or thinking what we are, do or think."[98] Critique attends in order to provoke us to look back at what sustains us and to speak out on its behalf. It aims toward Peter Buffet's urgent call to disturb "our current structures and systems," if not "shatter" them, in order to live differently by deferring to the incandescent signs of life. Foucault frequently reminds the reader that Man and modernity still inscribe our own horizon.[99]

For the attitude of modernity, the high value of the present is indissociable from a desperate eagerness to imagine it, to imagine it otherwise than it is, and to transform it "not by destroying it but by grasping it in what it is." Baude-lairean modernity is "an exercise in which extreme attention to what is real is confronted with the practice of a liberty that simultaneously respects this reality and violates it."[100]

Commenting on Baudelaire and *dandysme*, Foucault argues that the task for "modern man" is not to liberate his natural being from repressive force but to "invent himself." As no tooth and claw predetermine his identity, man must "produce" himself. Martin Heidegger's *Being and Time* and Jean-Paul Sartre's *Being and Nothingness*, two canonical texts of high modernism, both locate man's essence in his being "a being whose being is in question."[101] More recently, Judith Butler has demonstrated the element of performativity and role of self-invention in identity.[102]

At the same time, Foucault identifies freedom with the "freedom *not* to be who I am." To the extent that the individual is defined as a member of a popu-lation, certain elements of destiny are predetermined. Women are, as women, likely to be underpaid relative to men and to do far more than their share of do-mestic tasks. They are overrepresented in low-wage service positions and more likely than men to be the victims of sexual and domestic violence. Black men in the United States are more likely to be the victims of violence than women or men of other races. They are also more likely to become targets of regular-ized violence (school guards, police, agents of incarceration). The children of the poor are more likely to be poor as adults. Any human would want the freedom to escape these probabilities that are prescribed by current infrastructures of ex-perience. No one wants to be treated as that woman or black man or child. No one wants to be underpaid or to be more likely than others to be incarcerated or murdered. No one wants to be chronically poor. These universals appear by thinking nonspeculatively as a body in the solidarity of bodies.

At the end of the eighteenth century, medicine was transformed when physi-cians "opened up a few corpses" to reveal the lesion of the disease. The "visibility of death" replaces the "metaphysics of evil." As the "concrete a priori of medi-cine," death does not indicate a corruption of nature, a "counter-nature"; rather, it "become[s] *embodied* in the *living bodies* of individuals." The anatomico-pathological method of modern medicine and its techniques and technology comprise the "armed, positive, full form of [man's] finitude." At this point, "medical thought is fully engaged in the philosophical status of man" because it provides the paradigm logical figure for the "sciences of man," where the universal appears on the basis of "his elimination."[103]

Death links the "universality of language" and the "precarious, irreplaceable form of the individual."[104] For my utterances to make sense, they must be repeatable by other possible speakers. Sense depends on my being subject to displacement. Language is universal because the narrative or nominative position does not belong to me alone, but circulates across a community of speakers. The utterance is detachable from the particular speaker and does not rely on her presence to make sense. It will still mean long after she is dead.[105]

Attending to sexual difference and women's experience, however, opens up another domain of universals, one not based on death but on the universal solidarity of bodies. My body has always already been inside someone else's and continuous with it. Individuals exist only as moments of relationships and are sustained by them. How might this intergenerational generativity and bodily solidarity inform ethics and politics? Solidarity resists the reduction of the living being to a case or a member of a population subject to displacement and disposition through the general name. When I learn of a rape, I understand the injustice in the possibilities of my own body. The rape of a woman cannot possibly be just: this is something universal. Cutting and mutilating healthy girls cannot possibly be just, anymore than teaching them to be ashamed of their bodies is consistent with respect for life. The material universal of a woman's body teaches me both the aim of generativity and the injustice of violence, shame, immobility, sexualization, and capitalization. Thinking through sexual difference and women's embodied experience produces *human* universals, solidarities based on life, not violence and the fear of death.

Every reader knows the joy of being left alone and lost in a book. This liberty has been denied to girls. Rousseau prescribes the necessity of interrupting girls absorbed in such pursuits in order to forestall the development of any sense, on their part, of being at liberty. The gender division of labor and the normative practices associated with it discourage or punish girls for enjoying their own intellectual curiosity, despite the fact that educating girls appears to promote community health and decrease violence. Sometimes girls face the Hester Prynne "shirt of shame"; sometimes girls face something far more sinister. Sometimes girls risk their lives to go to school, just as in the antebellum South of the United States a slave risked being whipped or lynched for teaching another slave to read.

In some parts of the world, violent proponents of sexual propriety and the gender division of labor prohibit girls' education. Under the Taliban in Afghanistan from 1996 to 2001, no girls attended school. In Afghanistan in 2008, nearly one-third of the 7 million children in school were girls. In November 2008 one of those schoolgirls, who had a right to her liberty, her curiosity, and her dreams, and several schoolmates were on their way to school when their bus was attacked. The assailants asked, "Are you on the way to school?" The men tore off Shamsia's veil and sprayed acid in her face. Such acid attacks on individuals are part of a well-orchestrated campaign that has included poisoning water and food supplies at girls' schools as well as attacking them with poison gas.

Shamsia Husseini recovered and returned to school, subsequently becoming a teacher of another wave of girls. Her own analysis of the event yields a sharp critique of gender and property as well as the apparatus of subjection. The people who did this to her, she said, want her to be a "stupid thing," not merely stupid but also a thing. Perhaps they have some clue that educating Shamsia Husseini may be just the thing to "shatter our current structures." A girl with a book transgresses both the law of property and the gender division of labor.

PART TWO

Refiguring Ethics

What characterizes power is the fact that it is a strategic relation which has been stabilized through institutions. So the mobility in power relations is limited, and there are strongholds that are very, very difficult to suppress because they have been institutionalized and are now very pervasive in courts, codes, and so on. All this means that the strategic relations of people are made rigid.

—MICHEL FOUCAULT, "SEX, POWER, AND
THE POLITICS OF IDENTITY" (1994)

We live in a relational world that institutions have considerably impoverished. Society and the institutions which frame it have limited the possibility of relationships because a rich relational world would be very complex to manage. We should fight against the impoverishment of the relational fabric.

—MICHEL FOUCAULT, "THE SOCIAL TRIUMPH
OF THE SEXUAL WILL" (1997)

It is better to have possibilities for the future than to be already totally determined by the past.

And, it is better, too, to remain living persons: men and women, than to become neutral, abstract, artificial individuals, members of a social machine which functions more or less efficiently, but with no possibility of being governed, and in which identity and relationships between persons come second to the rule of money and to the arbitrary authority of certain decisions.

—LUCE IRIGARAY, "A TWO-SUBJECT CULTURE" (1994)

HUMANBODIES ARE ALWAYS already dependent on the ones who came before, on the mother, on those who labored to produce food and to secure potable water, on those who built infrastructures of roads or railways to sustain mobility or infrastructures of energy that light the world, provide heat in cold weather, and power all the machineries of modern life. Every humanbody is dependent on her teachers and on those who came before and created enterprises wherein she can find a living.

Relationships have long been mediated by money, but, at the end of the eighteenth century, human relations—among humans, with other animals, and with Earth—are increasingly subject to the logic of capital and corporate interests in population wealth.[1] Already for Hobbes, human relationships were determined by the exchange of signs of power: the worth of an individual is determined by his value on the market, by his "Price, that is to say so much as would be given for the use of his Power."[2] Under capital, however, the logic of the market extends throughout his experience, at the same time that the homogeneous scale of money overrides and masters all other signs of power. In this "relational world," no relation remains private and uncommodified, and no system of signs resists translation into the calculations of money.[3] Virtually everything is for sale, and anything—a child, a kidney, a car, an ice cream—is evaluated on the same scale: how much does it cost? Individuals live in a culture of possibilities that subordinates affective life to cost-benefit analysis. Economists, for example, regularly calculate the "cost" of having a child.[4] While parents anguish over the cost of a child's education, a precondition for his economic productivity, children anguish over the economic burden of their aging parents. Intergenerational generativity itself has been permeated by the figures of conceptualization, sexualization, and capitalization that serve population wealth.

What relationships are possible, what degree of fluidity and generativity can be enjoyed in relationships, depends not only on institutions, codes, and laws but also on the images and narratives that sustain them. This capitalization of relationships goes hand in hand with their sexualization, their *oedipalization*. If Freud installed the oedipal narrative as the template of personal identity, a hundred years earlier Hegel had already instituted the oedipal family as the infrastructure of ethics and politics. In Hegel's analysis, ethical life first appears in the figure of Antigone, who adheres to the *claim of the right* and provides a critical phenomenology of the "moral insolence" of reason. Antigone introduces the gender division of labor that will define both the good, or the ethics of family life, and justice, or the politics of public life. Through her service to her father or brother, caring for his body, a woman frees Man for science, politics, war, and philosophy. The gender division of labor solves the material problem, one that cannot be ignored for long, of how to integrate the demands of public and private generativity, work and family.

Critical phenomenology attends to the interface of words and bodies, where images and narratives inform experience. It aims to make the familiar strange so as to open up the possibility of (not) being who we are.

With regard to the oedipal family, it is important to remember that *it is only a play*.

There are other stories.

3

Antigone and Ismene

HARD HEADS, HARD HEARTS, AND
THE CLAIM OF THE RIGHT

A stubborn daughter of a stubborn sire.

—CHORUS, *ANTIGONE*, L. 471

No fool . . . like the obstinate fool.

—TIRESIAS, *ANTIGONE*, L. 1027

You've sent the one who should be among the living to the dead, and left the dead among the living.

—TIRESIAS, *ANTIGONE*, LL. 1068–69

What would my life be without you?

—ISMENE TO ANTIGONE, *ANTIGONE*, L. 548

AS DERRIDA ARGUES, the Hegelian text *must* be read.[1] Feminist philosophers have confirmed this imperative. Political philosophers and theorists who begin from the necessity of thinking through the problem of gender regularly find Hegel's account of the character of Antigone from Sophocles' eponymous play to be required reading.[2] Despite important diversities of position, these thinkers—Benhabib and Butler or Irigaray and Patricia Mills, for example—are virtually unanimous in their reading of Antigone's character on three points of analysis that are decisive for politics and philosophy.

For these readers, Antigone constitutes a *heroic* figure. She provides a new paradigm of feminist agency against the passivity normally assigned to women and reputedly exhibited by her little sister Ismene. Seyla Benhabib, like most feminist commentators, explicitly identifies Antigone as a model of feminist civil disobedience, an agency unafraid to risk itself against power on behalf of what is right.[3] These readers identify heroism with Antigone's willingness to risk her life, and they admire her for this detachment from life.

Second, these feminist readers identify both Antigone's heroism and her role in Hegel's text with her opposition to the state on behalf of the claims of blood relationship and family ties. They read Hegel as attempting to subordinate the family to the state, just as Creon did, and argue that Antigone not only represents the integrity of the feminine domain of the family but also a point of critique in Hegel's plan to install the hegemony of the modern nation-state over this realm.[4]

Third, these readers agree that Antigone is a transgressive figure: she transgresses not only the limits of the family as enforced by the state, and the difference between kinship and law, but also the difference of gender itself. This account of transgression understands gender and normalizing force—the laws of property as they apply to human bodies and the disciplines of sexual propriety— as effects of *patriarchy* and valorize Antigone as if she were an effective agent of its disruption.

Indeed, in this reading Antigone is *doubly* transgressive: within patriarchy taken as the infrastructure of women's subjected and confined agency and within Hegel's text itself, where the very agency he ascribes to Antigone appears to subvert the gender logic he means to install as absolutely necessary. Antigone transgresses both patriarchy and Hegel's thought by transgressing gender itself, and it is this gesture that secures her heroic stature in these feminist readings.

Both Benhabib and Butler describe Antigone as "masculine." Benhabib follows Schlegel in reading her as an "androgynous ideal" who "combines the male and female personality." She "transcends stereotypes and represents a blending of male and female characteristics."[5] Butler goes so far as to say that "in some sense" Antigone "is a man."[6] She transgresses the difference between public and private by transgressing gender, by claiming the agency of a man and deploying it against the state in the name of the family.[7]

A final point of agreement within this community of readers concerns the character of Ismene. Against this reading of Antigone as both heroic guardian of the family and fearless transgressor of gender difference, almost ubiquitous among feminist commentators, her little sister Ismene appears to represent a "merely feminine" position,[8] passive and incapable of the agency and self-determination exhibited by Antigone. Commentators frequently sneer at her, just as Antigone does in the play. She is cowardly, merely attached to the living body, and unwilling to risk her life for what is right.[9]

Patricia Mills gives Ismene unusual mention in her excellent essay "Hegel's *Antigone*."[10] Mills takes Ismene as a figure of "sisterly solidarity." Unlike the heroic Antigone who valorizes the attachment to her brother, Ismene roots her sense of the right and of the familial claim in the sister–sister relation. Mills observes that Hegel "completely disregards this aspect of the play."[11]

Mills, however, goes on to disregard it herself in favor of the conventional rendering of Ismene as passively determined by the materialities of life. She quickly dismisses Ismene from the scene of political theory, relegating her to the position of the "traditional woman." Mills argues that Ismene "wavers in her commitment to the good" and that, in "siding with the law of the polis," she "bows to male domination." Her reading reinforces Antigone's figuration as the heroic transgressor of gender arrangements who "refuses to fit neatly into Hegel's system."[12]

One might wonder why, against the competing claim of the living sister, the sacrifice for the dead brother constitutes a "commitment to the good," rendering Antigone heroic. One might wonder why abandoning the living sister in order to die for the dead brother should command respect.

DEATH IS WOMAN'S WORK

This reading of Antigone as the heroine of family ties and / or gender complexity misreads both Sophocles' trilogy and Hegel's reading of it in ways that undermine feminism itself. Not only do these readings ignore Ismene's own agency within the text, they also fail to appreciate the way in which Antigone's action turns away from life and sisterly solidarity in favor of fraternity and its assignment of women to the care of the body.[13] This heroic reading of Antigone, central to feminism and feminist political theory, in fact reinscribes the very infrastructures of subjection that it means to disrupt and dismantle.

First, Antigone represents precisely those kinship structures that install woman as the paradigm of property, the original medium of a *fraternal* exchange. This traffic in women elaborates and sustains the lateral relations of fraternity wherein patriarchy itself is sustained.[14] The security and authority of patriarchal structures depends on the father's membership in the civil and political structures of fraternity.[15] Hobbes' "little Monarch" only enjoys his dominion over the little kingdom of his subjects, his wife, children, and servants, because his brothers, the other men in his horizon, recognize his right to rule in his family, as he recognizes their right to rule in theirs. It is his status as a citizen among his fellow citizens that secures Man's dominion in his own property, including his women and children.

In Hegel's analysis, women are twice subjected: once in the family and again in the state. Antigone represents not only a woman's duty to her "little Monarch" but also the subjection of women's bodies and generativity to the fraternal order. She is both the "guardian of the blood" and the one who supplies the flesh and blood necessary to sustain the fraternal economy.[16] At once the paradigm of property, a capitalized generativity, and the source of domestic labor, women's bodies generate and sustain the brother's bonds.

Second, feminism's reading of Antigone as heroic reinforces Hegel's assignment to women, as their essential work, the task of sustaining the body. The purpose and result of this labor is to *free* man *from* the body and its needs, so that he may be *free for* the theoretical pursuits of politics and science. By tending to her aged father, Antigone frees her brothers for their military and political pursuits, as the play explicitly notes.[17] Her labor belongs to and sustains male agency, as well as the system of fraternal relations in which man's disputes over property are negotiated and the resources of the family put into circulation.

Third, far from subverting or disturbing the distinction of public and private, Antigone is complicit with the very material, legal, and normative structures that enforce the division of life into public and private, state and family, a community of laws and a tribe of blood relations. It is Creon, as the power of the state, who violates this difference through the improper interference in what should have been a family matter. By stubbornly sticking to his stupid decree, denying the family and private life its own integrity and independence from the administrative and regulatory power of the state, Creon puts the entire community in danger.

Hegel's analysis does not advance the prerogatives of the state at the expense of the family, as these feminist readings regularly assert; rather, it is just the state's failure to recognize the integrity of the family sphere and its practices that is at issue in his reading. The family embodies a set of essential sustaining powers, just as the state does, and each is compromised when one assumes the prerogatives of the other. For Hegel, the Oedipus cycle is not an occasion to assert the authority of the state over the family, but a demonstration of the disastrous consequences for both the state and the family when the two are confused.

The Oedipal cycle presents a state no less subjected to the family than the family is to it. For Hegel, such confusion always produces tribalism, factionalism, and terrorism. Where the power of judicial authority is concentrated in the family, there are inevitably wars of succession as well as wars among families. Tribalism is synonymous with the state of war as Hobbes defined it: "So the nature of War consisteth not in actual fighting, but in the known disposition therein, during all the time there is no assurance to the contrary."[18] Ancient and recent history, whether in Europe or Asia or Africa, demonstrates with painful clarity how a political structure that places authority in tribal elders also renders women property and war a way of life. Injuries are crimes against the blood and must be paid with blood. Men are massacred and their women systematically raped to eliminate a rival tribe.[19] Schoolgirls are kidnapped and sold or awarded serially as "wives" to be raped repeatedly by murderous extremists whose name positions an opposition to educating girls at the center of their violent agenda.[20] A woman is publicly raped by a rival family to pay for her brother's alleged impertinence.[21] Around the globe where tribalism—the confusion of family and state—persists, differences of blood and histories of vengeance make futures impossible.

Antigone belongs to this state of war. While the brother leaves the family behind for politics, science, and war, she remains assigned to the family and its specific labor. Its labor, in contrast to the work that defines the public domains of the state, science, and philosophy, concerns the dead as much as the living: Antigone's action installs the burial of the dead body as the paradigm of women's work. Her agency not only reinforces the division between man's formative activity in the public sphere and the privacy of female agency but also identifies the latter not with the generativity of childbearing but with the theatrical performance of the burial rite. While the purpose of the rite may be to respiritualize the dead body, what the performance actually produces is the mere representation of the (dead) other, who has become an impossible presence.

In death the body has become a thing like any other, subject to alien forces. The crows pick at its eyes and the worms attack its flesh.[22] The burial rite represents the corpse as if the dead body were still a member of the community, as if it were still animated by the narrative force proper to it, *as if it were alive after death*, as if Antigone's actions after his death could matter to Polyneices himself. Though she is destined to care for the body while it is alive, the limit of woman's responsibility lies in these concrete practices through which the (dead) other is ritually remembered so as to be re-membered and reinstalled in the community.

It is not for the corpse, however, for what Polyneices has become, that the act has results. An actual transubstantiation takes place in which the living flesh of Polyneices becomes the dead thing, the corpse. Nothing can ever again matter to Polyneices. Antigone may say she acts for Polyneices, but it is her promise that remains, and, as she acknowledges, it is to be true to herself and her own life that she buries him.[23]

Moreover, everyone has a stake in the burial practices, for, as Theseus reflects, "I know myself a mortal, and can hope for no more in the end than you can" (l. 568). The stark fact that one day *you* will be the putrescent, worm-ridden corpse, unless your bones are first picked clean by dogs and crows, motivates mysterious machineries of salvation and transubstantiation. The funeral rites may be mere representations, but they sustain not the dead other but the community itself by protecting its members from the stark terror of an irreducible mortality, from the stark knowledge that one will eventually, sooner or later, be the body filled with worms.

Hegel takes religion and its artifacts to be one more historical formation, one more set of practices by which the sociality of human life is sustained. While announcing the philosophical necessity of thinking human mortality without compensation, Hegel nonetheless admits the practical necessity of social mechanisms for managing death, for, so to speak, not everyone is a philosopher. Thus, Antigone is involved in what for Hegel is a kind of noble lie. The funeral rites effectively address the community's loss and, more importantly, forestall a real confrontation with mortality by representing the dead other as respiritualized and restored.[24]

This exorcism of death, this representation of the dead body as if it were still alive, defines Antigone, just as it is the definitive task of woman. Woman's management of death, the rites and practices through which the corpse is respiritualized for the community, prove essential to sustaining the human community, as they make it possible for the individual to believe that there is some compensation for his own death.[25] Through the funeral rite for the dead other, the living member of the community identifies with the continuity of the blood and the community that will survive him. His confidence in the funeral rite relieves the warring brother of any anxiety about the dishonoring of his dead body. Neither tending the living body—caring for children, the infirm, and the elderly—nor tending the dead body in the funeral rite will yield the reciprocity of mutual recognition that Man enjoys in politics and science.

Woman constitutes for Hegel the "eternal irony of the community" because she is at once absolutely necessary to its life and formally excluded from participating in it. The brothers depend upon her to tend the body and the blood, and they find the moment of life preserved for themselves in her. This is no mere metaphorical dependence, but a material dependence of Man on woman's unpaid (or underpaid) labor in the private sphere where bodies are maintained.

The relation, as Irigaray points out, is not reciprocal. In Hegel's analysis, the figures of mother and wife are always objectified by a natural desire. The brother represents, as Irigaray remarks, a "possibility of recognition of which she is deprived as mother and wife."[26] The brother-sister relation seems to offer woman a possibility of recognition as a subject, insofar as it is not determined by the desire for her body. Even if one accepts this story of the brother-sister relation as innocent of carnal desire, the sister cannot find herself as a discursive subject realized and sustained in her brother's experience. The gender division of labor and the assignment of woman to materiality and the body deprive her of the detachment necessary to mutual recognition. She cannot return his gaze of recognition: she cannot see herself in his pursuits as he can see himself in her milieu of bodily need, even as he detaches from it. As she is excluded from participation in his arenas of action, she is inadequate in herself to reflect the brother's agency. She can only "devote herself to his cult after death."[27] Incapable of returning his gaze so as to complete the circuit of mutual recognition necessary to establish her as a subject, she remains subjected to the body and its care.

That devotion, however, derives from the need of the *living* brother and from Antigone's own promise to him. A soldier, all too familiar with the dogs and crows of the battlefield, Polyneices is anxious to be relieved of his worry over his dead body, as he actively imagines his death. He appeals to both sisters and presses Antigone in particular to unburden him of its care, claiming her, not once but twice, by her duty toward his dead body.[28] Just as the funeral rite serves the community, staving off the terror of mortality and repairing the breach in social bonds created by the impossible presence of the (dead) other, so too Antigone's devotion begins before death, when her troubled brother relieves his mind by reminding her of her duty to him. Women's labor preserves the moment of life for a man, so that he may be freed for thought and war.

While each man transcends himself in the fraternity of citizens, in the generalized figure of the citizen, no such infrastructure of transcendence exists for women.[29] Her participation in the discursive domains of science, politics, and philosophy, Hegel insists, "puts these domains themselves in danger."[30] There will be exceptions. Some women will be capable of these pursuits; however, their entry into these domains jeopardizes the entire human enterprise by leaving the body untended. In Hegel's analysis this commitment to the body in life and in death prohibits woman from participating in the collaborative enterprises of science, politics, and philosophy, where she might experience herself, as a man does, as a moment of something universal. The funeral rite is something universal, but, unlike war or science, it is a spectacle with no formative result in the world of action that might reflect her agency, expand the culture of possibilities, and provide for new opportunities for action. The funeral rites can only be repeated, and a woman's agency belongs to the invisibility of the "netherworld."[31] The community depends upon her actual generativity, while, ironically, she is assigned to the symbolic performance of the rites of death.

In Hegel's analysis, Antigone figures not only the necessity of this difference as the material infrastructure of community but also the *immediacy* of the claim of the right. In his reading, her heroic status depends not on her adherence to the family against the state but on her demonstration of the origin of duty in social relationships rather than in the abstract arguments of reason. Hegel founds ethics on this phenomenology of the way in which a woman discovers herself to be always already bound by certain commitments. She is always already faced with actions that *must be done*. Human beings find themselves ethically claimed in the experience of being mother, son, or daughter. Polyneices claims her promise *as her brother,* and she gives it *as his sister*. No argument is required to establish the duty of caring for a child or an aged parent; rather, the reverse is true: an argument is required to justify the failure to do so. One of the chief phenomenological features of mothering is the sense of necessity in ordinary quotidian tasks: children must be fed. Antigone represents the immediacy and sociality of being claimed by the right as over against the interiority of virtue or the abstractness of law.[32] The individual exists only as a node in a network of relations where ethical obligation is always already in place, preceding and informing reflection.

Locating ethical obligation in the primacy of social relations, Hegel decries the moral "insolence" of reason in making obligation contingent upon its own test.[33] Such a philosophical gesture divests the right of its force of command. Hegel remarks that "it would be strange" if the law of noncontradiction, which establishes only the formal limits of theoretical or mathematical truth, were to yield a greater result in the area of practical action.[34] The test of universalizability, he argues, "fits every case equally well, and is thus in fact no criterion at all."[35] The law of property is no more self-consistent than the idea of ownership in common, just as an individual, without contradicting himself, can give his property to another so that it becomes the other's. Hegel notes that the reverse process, whereby an individual comes to see as his own something that has been entrusted to him by another, is no less consistent.

> It is not, therefore, because I find something is not self-contradictory that it is right; on the contrary, it is right because it is what is right. That something is the property of another, this is fundamental; I have not to argue about it, or hunt around for or entertain thoughts, connections, aspects, of various kinds: I have to think neither of making laws nor of testing them . . . since if I liked, I could in fact just as well make the opposite conform to my indeterminate tautological knowledge and make *that* the law. . . . I could make whichever of them I liked the law, and just as well neither of them, and as soon as I start to test them I have already begun to tread an unethical path.[36]

In this analysis of the limits of law as a concept in ethics, Hegel's critique of the law of property exposes its contingency. In this passing example, Hegel gives the game away. He repeats the same impossible relation between reason and nature that Hobbes installed. The law of property is not rational because it is established by reason but because it is required by Man's nature. His dissociative nature requires the law for his survival, and the first law of nature and of reason is that a rational animal cannot act contrary to his own self-interest. Reason establishes itself against nature, immediacy, and animal interest as abstraction, deferral, and displacement. Yet what animates reason, without which it would be an inert formula, an "empty husk," is animal interest, and what installs the law of property and sexual propriety as its first principle is Man's violently competitive nature.

This, however, is not all that nature teaches. Perhaps women and children, who always seem to appear in the plural, unlike Man, provide a different figure, more like the sociable bees. Perhaps there are other girls than these wretched sisters, girls who play, beyond Rousseau's injunctions, in a meadow of flowers. Though Hegel's analysis does not investigate these story lines, it does recognize, in the valorization of Antigone's devotion, that ethics begins with the immediate experience of my dependency on the other and the other's dependency on me, not with a test meant to preserve reason's own purity or self-consistency. Reason's attempt to make the right contingent upon its own test divests the right of its power to command. This "unethical path" leads away from the sociality of ethical life.

This heroic moment in Hegel's reading of Antigone, however, is qualified by an equally profound moment of critique. As Tiresias counsels Creon, "Stubbornness and stupidity are twins."[37] What distinguishes the entire Cadmean clan for Hegel is the double tendency to issue unilateral, peremptory decisions and then to stick to them with absolute fixity. Antigone exhibits the same "stubbornness" that proves the downfall of Creon, her brothers, and her father himself. Like Creon, Antigone is guilty of the *hardheadedness* of sticking to one moment of the right at the expense of the other and of the *hardheartedness* of elevating abstract principles over living social relations. This hardness, a kind of ethical immobility, is the ethical equivalent of the epistemological error of "natural consciousness" who regularly takes the part for the whole or sticks doggedly to one side of an essential distinction at the expense of the other. This immobility or rigidity can be sustained only at the expense of the fluidity of experience where bodies, like thoughts, are meant to be motile, moving.

Against the purity and self-consistency of reason's "beautiful soul," Antigone exhibits, in Hegel's reading, the way in which valid moral claims inevitably conflict. To act is to be guilty, Hegel argues: "Innocence, therefore, is merely non-action, like the mere being of a stone, not even that of a child."[38] You are a young mother and a teacher. Your aged mother, who lives hundreds of miles away, falls ill. What do you do? Do you leave your family and students to care for her? Life frequently presents claims that cannot be successfully negotiated without leaving some valid claims only partially addressed or even unanswered. To be human is to be in need of forgiveness and to need to be forgiving.

Antigone acts as she does because she has been claimed: Polyneices specifically charges her with his care after death. The destruction that results from her action does not call into question the legitimacy of the claim, but reflects her stubborn hardheartedness in adhering to it, given the cost in lives, including her own. By acting to honor the obligation that Polyneices, not once but twice, lays on her, she abandons her sister, her future husband, and her own life.[39] She might have done it quietly or without owning the deed, but, by abandoning all other obligations, by rigidly sticking to one at the expense of all others, refusing to move between them and negotiate among them, she brings destruction on herself and her family.

Feminism's failure to criticize Antigone and its mistaken attribution to Hegel of a dismissal of the family in favor of the state make it susceptible to the same hardheadedness and hardheartedness that Hegel criticizes in Antigone and Creon.[40] The heroic figuration of Antigone reinscribes the opposition between the family and state that is called into question by Hegel's critique and forestalls any attempt to reimagine a politics of the body not already informed by Man's gender norms.[41]

The division of gender is for Hegel essentially a division of *labor*. Woman's work in caring for the dead body is as essential to the maintenance of the fraternal economy as is her service to the needs of the living body, and by valorizing

Antigone's action feminist readers reinscribe this material logic of life and death, becoming complicit in its sacrifice of actual life to speculative abstraction.

Lacking a material infrastructure of transcendence, lacking access to the institutions of collaboration and solidarity in science, politics, and philosophy, women remain tied to the particularity of the body and blood relationship. In Hegel's analysis, woman is, as Irigaray remarks, the "lining of man's coat," the complement to Man produced by Rousseau's educational regimen.[42] Feminism's heroic Antigone reinforces the very system of gender installed by Hegel's text, those pervasive normative arrangements organized by the difference between men and women's labor.[43]

ISMENE RUNS AROUND

In spite of the hypervaluation of this oedipal narrative, by Hegel and feminist philosophers alike, it is not clear why feminist readers, or indeed any reader, should consider a character heroic who abandons her living sister in favor of her dead brother. Why should we affirm with Irigaray and other readers Antigone's relation to her mother as mediated by the brother and not her sister?[44] Equally as important, why should the mother's love be prejudged as a form of sexual desire whose logic is always already marked masculine, a marking constantly reinforced by psychoanalysis?

Hegel's reading of *Antigone* is the starting point for his constant condemnation of the fixed unyielding mind. In his analysis the play reveals the evil done by a precipitous, unilateral judgment lacking the fluidity necessary to mediate among all the elements of the right. Yet feminist commentators regularly misread Hegel so as to miss entirely Antigone's role in his argument, both as avatar of the right and as paradigm of the selfish rigidity that undermines thought, action, and solidarity. This hardheadedness and hardheartedness oppose life and generativity.

Feminist commentators deride Ismene as the necessary inverse to the glorification of Antigone that so misreads her character and Hegel's reading of it. To represent Ismene as a "caricature" of the feminine in virtue of "her weakness, her fear, her submissive obedience, her tears, madness, hysteria," is, however, simply not to read the plays.[45] Far from Antigone being an exception to the usual Cadmean hardheadedness and hardheartedness, she adheres strictly to the gender division of labor, even as she sacrifices the future to the dead. Ismene, on the other hand, always acts for the future and to promote life. She is the only Cadmean who exhibits the fluidity of thought and feeling that Hegel associates with philosophy and ethical life. Oedipus, Antigone, Creon, Polyneices, and Eteocles all childishly indulge themselves in precipitous pronouncements to which they cling with unrelenting stubbornness, in spite of the destruction that their hardheadedness and hardheartedness wreak on their family and community. Ismene alone substitutes effective negotiation and tireless efforts at reconciliation for the petulant selfishness and intransigence of her family. She repeatedly exhibits not only enormous courage, loyalty, and reliability but also an ability to keep her head while the rest of the Cadmeans, most especially Antigone, are losing theirs and bringing on the destruction of all.

Psychoanalysis has so infected the plays with the masculine logic of desire, possession, and surveillance to which it would reduce all pleasure and all life that it is almost impossible to read them otherwise. Still, one only has to resist the elision of the middle play, which these commentators rarely touch upon and Freud ignores altogether, to see that neither the reduction of the play to a psychological trope nor the glorification of Antigone's hardheadedness and hardheartedness can be sustained.

Throughout *Oedipus at Colonus*, Ismene keeps her head and acts on behalf of others. Ismene exhibits an ability and a willingness to listen that is anything but passive. Rather than precipitously expressing herself in some commandment that inflicts harm on all, even as it realizes the egoism of the one who pronounces it, Ismene listens *as a prelude to action*. By listening, she understands what must be done in order to appease the conflicting claims of the right, and she is ready to collaborate with others in order to secure the future. Mobility of person, mobility of ideas and perspective, the capacity to negotiate among conflicting claims, and the inclination to listen to others and to forge collaborations prior to action define Ismene's courage and heroism against the cruel and futile willfulness of Antigone. Her mobility of person, thought, and feeling allows her alone among the Cadmean clan to exceed both the gender division of labor and the unrelenting fixity of thought and will that makes any future impossible.

In *Oedipus at Colonus* Oedipus regularly treats the two sisters as a pair, referring to them equally as "my props," entreating them to "press me close on either side."[46] Throughout the play, both sisters command respect as supplements to his impaired agency, though it is Ismene who serves as his executor among political and religious powers, while Antigone performs the feminine labor of caring for his body. Both are equally distraught at the death of their father. Even Antigone, who in the next play will set up the dismissive interpretations that have crowded around her sister, identifies her own devotion to her father as no greater than Ismene's.[47] In this play, Antigone celebrates not the hardheaded hardheartedness of virtue but the sisterly solidarity she has shared with Ismene, a solidarity that has sustained them both.

Of the two sisters it is Ismene, however, not Antigone, who is the active force in *Oedipus at Colonus.* Ismene comes on the scene as a figure of agency or mobility, a bold figure of strength and courage who, like Hermes or Dionysus, transgresses gender norms. She plays the dangerous role of a double agent at Thebes, serving, as Oedipus remarks, as his "faithful agent" or "outpost," who "eludes the Cadmeans vigilance."[48] Oedipus emphasizes the integrity of her agency, remarking that it is Ismene herself who has had the wit and courage to establish herself as his "agent." Her actions are neither prescribed by the codes of gender nor the result of another's instruction. The representation of Ismene as slavish, overly attached to life, or unwilling to risk her life for what is right can be read into the last play only by ignoring the second one. So far from being "weak," "typically feminine," or "hysterical," Ismene exhibits rare courage and intelligence by operating effectively under surveillance, in hostile territory, even as she violates in every register the boundaries that define gender norms.

In order to convey what she considers crucial intelligence, she eludes Creon's surveillance and steals away from Thebes in search of her father and sister. After an arduous and treacherous journey, she discovers them at the sanctuary near Athens. Ismene arrives, almost unrecognized by Antigone, astride "a colt of Aetna's breed."[49] She wears no mere "sun hat," as some translators imply, but a hat that was both a traveling garment, indicating that Ismene had come a long way, and a warrior's helmet. The *petasos* or Thessalian hat is regularly associated with the liberty of mobility and the ability to cross borders. It is the hat not only of travelers but also of Hermes, the peripatetic god of borders and messages. Like Hermes, Ismene fearlessly traverses the boundaries, both literal and

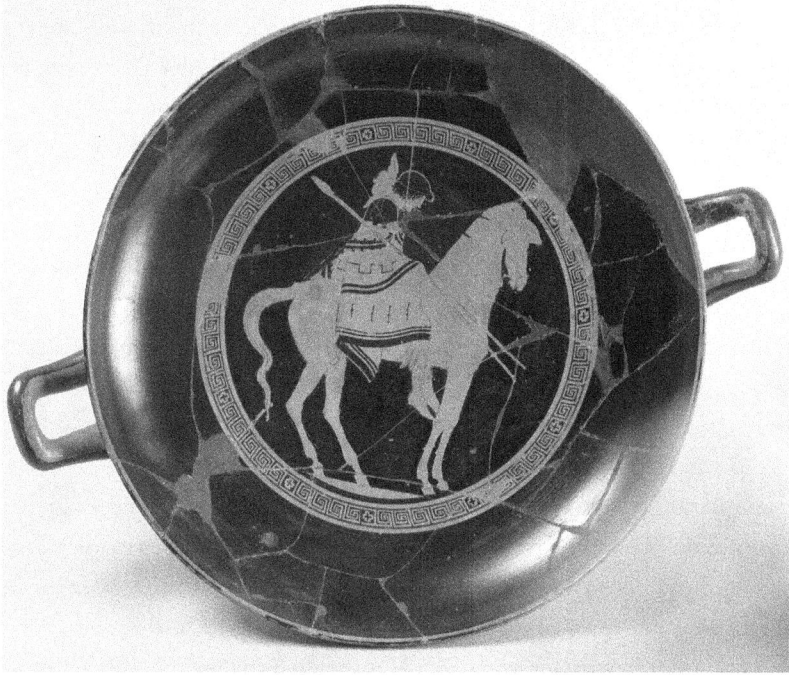

FIGURE. 3.1. Attic red-figure cup depicting a rider on horseback. Euphronios (fl. ca. 520–500 B C, workshop of). Musée du Louvre, Paris, France / Bridgman Images

figurative, that are laid down for her in order to serve as the conduit among conflicting powers as well as the point of their negotiation. Ismene does not stay home as girls and women are meant to do; she roams around at will in an effort to make peace among the powers that have assailed and continue to menace her family. In her physical and intellectual mobility, Ismene presents a new figure of women's agency beyond the gender logic of Man's law of property.

The *petasos* also invokes the courage of the warrior. On the famous Pergamon frieze in Berlin, a mounted youth wielding a spear wears this same "Thessalian hat."[50] The *petasos* was worn by Athenian youth when serving in the cavalry.[51] Through this hat and her entrance astride a noble steed, Winckelman identifies Ismene with a "mounted Amazon, contending with two warriors" depicted on an antique earthenware vessel as well as with numerous images of "Pallas the huntress."[52]

In contrast to Antigone, however, Ismene's courage is not self-aggrandizing. In the third play, Antigone is less focused on burying Polyneices, which might have been done quietly and in secret, than in proclaiming against Creon the glory of her virtue in doing so. Her actions have no other end than fulfilling the promise to the dead brother and indulging her own willful adherence to the virtue of her deed above any other value. Hobbes remarks that the third cause of war, after mastery and security, is "glory." In the first case men go to war to make themselves "master of other men's person, wives, children, and cattle"; in the second, to defend what they already possess. Those who quarrel over glory go to war over "trifles."[53] The brothers fight over property, but Antigone risks her life for an abstract value and her own glory. Hers is a nihilistic courage that serves the dead and her own death.[54] Perhaps there is a moment when she mourns the loss of the future, but she has no patience and never considers that she might be rescued. She leaves the food untouched and cuts off her own breath because she has no commitment to life. Ismene, on the other hand, acts always in the name of the future. In *Oedipus at Colonus* her life-threatening duplicity and running around serve only to negotiate between the conflicting powers. Just as in the third play, where her arguments both with Antigone and Creon focus on the future, here too she courageously risks her life to prevent further destruction and find a way forward for her family. Why should Antigone's pose as the guardian of virtue command admiration, as if the abstract principle were worth more than her courageous little sister?[55]

While Antigone bears his *body*, it is Ismene who helps Oedipus bear his *fate*. Antigone performs a typically feminized form of care in ministering to the body of her father and remaining by his side as his "support." Ismene serves her father through an agency that transgresses the norms of containment defining the feminine gender. It is Ismene who is sent by Oedipus to perform the sacrifice, of which he is physically incapable, that will ensure his hospitable welcome in the precinct of the Furies, while Antigone remains with him. And, it is Ismene who conjures for Oedipus his posthumous revenge, as his Theban kin, standing near his grave, find themselves engulfed by the miasma of his anger. In negotiating the claims of the political, religious, and familial authorities determining her family's fate, she proves herself to be not only a secure messenger but also a source of reliable interpretation and wise counsel.[56] She accurately assesses the intentions of Creon and her brothers, even as she assists Oedipus in interpreting the oracles. She counsels not only Antigone, but also both her brothers and her father, as well as Creon, to relent from their hardheadedness and hardheartedness. Ismene negotiates both human law and divine power with equal efficacy.

Arriving on her noble steed, capped for travel and war, Ismene has already shown her mettle as an undercover agent. Antigone has wandered with her father, ministering personally to his immediate bodily needs and sharing his sorrows. In doing so, she adheres to the gender division of labor by sticking to her domestic tasks and remaining within the precincts of the fraternal logic. Ismene, on the other hand, is a mobile agent, constantly transgressing domestic borders. Though she acts on behalf of others, her agency arises from her own initiative, ingenuity, and courage, as well as her desire to secure the future of her family and community.

The rest of the Cadmean clan follows the same script of hardheadedness and hardheartedness. Make a rash pronouncement without any consultation. Stick to it stubbornly *as a matter of principle,* in spite of wise counsel and the catastrophic consequences to which the decree dooms your family and your state. Ismene alone exhibits a generous fluidity of thought and feeling that makes her an effective agent among conflicting powers. Her agency is compromised only through the loss of her mobility when she is abducted by Creon in an attempt to gain leverage over her father. She is the first sister to be imprisoned, captured while on the move on her father's behalf.

In *Antigone,* when Creon seeks to establish his authority and to subjugate the sisters, he specifically contrasts the containment that he means to impose upon them with the freedom to "roam at large" that Ismene has exhibited, decreeing, "They must be women now. No more running around."[57]

ISMENE'S ETHICS OF LIFE: MOBILITY, FORGIVENESS, NEGOTIATION

In the third play, Ismene, so far from losing her head in hysteria or dissolving in fear, boldly argues with Creon on behalf of her sister: "Will you kill your own son's promised bride?"[58] She courageously appeals to Creon not to sacrifice his own future by sacrificing Antigone, a cost he pays for no better reason than to secure himself against a threat he had himself created.[59] She appeals not only for

Antigone's life but to the future and life itself as a value. The chorus repeats and authorizes her plaintive inquiry. Ismene argues on behalf of Antigone, not by justifying her action according to some calculus or procedure of reason but by invoking the future life that Antigone promises to her family and her city.

Most important, however, she makes a direct appeal to her sister to choose life with her over a sacrifice to the dead brother. She pleads with Antigone at the opening of the third play not to persist in her fatal course. Though Antigone, like most readers, immediately interprets her resistance as base cowardice, Ismene takes no offense. The scene ends with her words of love for her sister.[60] Given that Ismene shows no fear of death when she tells Creon that she wishes to share Antigone's fate, a more plausible interpretation of this passage would not ignore Ismene's surprise and alarm at Antigone's plan, nor her earnest effort to dissuade her sister. While there is still a chance of turning Antigone from this deadly purpose, Ismene will not join her in it. When the deed is done and Antigone condemned, Ismene is ready to stand by her side. "What could life offer me when you are gone?" she asks.[61] If the sisters experienced a new terror after the death of their father, when his presence and the need to care for him no longer obscured the horror of their circumstance, how much more awful will it be for the sister who finds herself all alone? For Ismene, the overriding value has always been her relations with the living, and particularly the living sister who has been her companion and collaborator in this long, lurid fate. Ismene, no less than Antigone, is "claimed by the right," but, rather than valorizing the abstraction of the dead body or the speculation of the funeral rite, she attends to the immediacy of the relation to the living sister.

Far from displaying cowardice, Ismene's trajectory in *Antigone* in relation to her sister exactly mirrors Antigone's own agency in relation to Polyneices in *Oedipus at Colonus*. Antigone makes every effort to dissuade Polyneices from the purpose to which he stupidly and stubbornly adheres in spite of certain disaster. The war is no less necessary to his identity than burying him is to Antigone's. Only when she realizes that she cannot turn him from this path does Antigone join him in his purpose by agreeing to bury him.[62] Similarly, Ismene, surprised and alarmed by her sister's plan, tries to dissuade Antigone, but when her failure to do so is clear, she attempts to join her sister in bearing the results of it. There was nothing cowardly in Antigone's effort to preserve the living relationship to her brother, just as there is nothing base in Ismene's identification of her own life with that of her living sister.

Antigone, however, like Polyneices, adheres to an abstract purpose over living relationships. Before Creon and the assembled multitude, Antigone, the hardhearted and hardheaded Cadmean, spurns her sister's attempt to join her as a partner in the deed. Before the city, Antigone laughs at Ismene and mocks her intentions. Still, the patient Ismene takes no offense. Ismene's response to this cruel public repudiation is to ask, "Is there some way I can help you even now?"[63] Inspired by her love of the living sister, she meets scorn with generosity.

Far from "siding with the polis," as Mills suggests, Ismene refuses to reject her sister, repeating to Creon, "What life would there be for me without my sister here?"[64] Why should we readers admire Antigone when she sneeringly spurns Ismene's solidarity as the impertinent intrusion of the weak willed into her noble purpose? Her action serves the fraternal economy and abandons the living sister. She puts the purity of her own conscience and adherence to an abstraction—for both the principle and the dead brother are abstractions—above the appeal of her living sister.

Ismene, on the other hand, will sacrifice any abstraction, for she values above all else the relation to the living sister. As she goes to her tomb, Antigone falters and laments that no one will mourn her. But, in offering to die with her, Ismene has already mourned Antigone: "What would my life be without you?"[65] Ismene has already imagined Antigone's death, and in so doing she has experienced life after the loss of her sister as unsustainable.[66] From the very beginning of *Antigone*, Ismene operates out of this sense of loss, of the catastrophic and irreversible transformation of the living sister into the impossible presence of the dead body.

Hegel's critical power is never more scathing than when applied to some logic of the beyond by which the truth of life and experience would be reduced in favor of an abstract concept. There is nothing beyond experience in Hegel's analysis, and the universal only appears in the immediacy of the actual human being and his works. Should a reader then be taken in by the representations of the funeral rites, as if the brother really were restored to the community, so that Antigone's sacrifice of her life and her abandonment of her sister might be justified? This logic of the beyond, of death, provides the infrastructure for the fraternal economy by which women are subjected.

The sisters reenact Hegel's famous drama of master and slave. Antigone, like the master, risks her life in order to prove her independence. Like the master, she proves to be a dead end.

Ismene, like the slave, is caught by an attachment to life in infrastructures of work and obedience. Perhaps, after a long struggle, she may yet free herself. Perhaps, after a long struggle, she may succeed in transforming these structures into a fabric that sustains each and all.

A CODA ON DEATH: BEYOND THE OEDIPAL FAMILY

In his analysis of *Antigone,* Hegel associates death with a divine law and the restoration of the community's loss through the respiritualization of the dead body in the funeral rite. Running throughout Sophocles' trilogy, however, is a persistent association of death, not with the illusionism of the funeral rite and a power beyond experience, but with mortality as a brute and unredeemable fact of life. In *Oedipus at Colonus* the aged Oedipus recites the immanence of death in life:

> To the gods alone
> Is given immunity from old age and death;
> Nothing else escapes the ruin of almighty time.
> Earth's powers waste away, the powers of men decay,
> Honor grows cold, dishonor flourishes,
> Little by little friendship wanes, between man and man,
> Between city and city, sooner or later,
> Pleasure sickens.[67]

A life encompasses, as both Proust and Hegel remark, many deaths of many selves. No compensation is offered in the play. Theseus emphasizes the intercalation of life and death in life: no one, not the young and healthy any more than the old and infirm, can avoid the immanence of death in life: "I know myself a mortal, and my share in what the morrow brings no more than thine."[68]

It is this difference between life and death that virtually all the characters restlessly negotiate. The plays are full of walking dead, of the living who wish to be dead, of the dead among the living and the living among the dead. Oedipus is a "breathing corpse." The living man Polyneices speaks in the name of his ghost in his last meeting with Antigone, while she openly mourns him as if he were already dead, just as Ismene mourns Antigone while she still lives. Tiresias warns Creon not to "kill the dead a second time" by prohibiting the burial of Polyneices. It is as if the unburied Polyneices still lives, or lives again, in the decisive effect that his unburied dead body has upon the living. Upon learning of Eurydice's suicide, Creon remarks, "I was dead, and you killed me again."[69] By confusing death and life, sending the living to die and leaving the dead among the living, Creon dooms himself and his city.[70]

In their exchange at the end of Oedipus at Colonus, both Antigone and Ismene express ambivalence in life because of an attachment to the dead. Ismene is the first to invite death to "take her breath" so that she might be delivered from a life of "desolation" in her father's absence. But Antigone makes the thought a plan: despite the injunction against it, she intends to visit her father's grave, and, when Ismene expresses concern, Antigone replies theatrically, foreshadowing her heroics in the next play, "Slay me!"

Deaths proliferate throughout these plays, as they do throughout Greek tragic drama. The cycle begins with a woman hanged and ends with a woman gored.[71] Antigone bemoans her fate at the end of Oedipus at Colonus: "Now we may weep indeed!" While Oedipus was alive, the sisters endured their fate "for his sake." After his death, when they are no longer occupied as his agent and caregiver, respectively, the sisters find themselves face-to-face with the "unrelenting horror" of their circumstance.[72] Jocasta cuts off her breath rather than live with this horror, just as Eurydice pierces her heart rather than live with the wound of her son's loss, who could not live with the stupid and unnecessary loss of Antigone, who did not wait for time to take her breath, so that the obstinate fool Creon was too late. Gory corpses pile up, and even the one left living, who now repents his stupidity and stubbornness, is "twice dead," having lost both his present (Eurydice) and his future (Haemon and Antigone).

The destruction derives from the oedipal temperament of hardheadedness and hardheartedness, as diagnosed for philosophy by Hegel, and of which only Ismene is an exception. Choleric, impatient, imperious and quick to judge, quick to blame others, stubborn, and not without a taste for revenge, from Cadmus to Pentheus to Oedipus, these guardians of virtue cannot be turned from their fixity of purpose. It is, after all, Oedipus himself who curses his sons rather than forgive them, sealing their violent fate, just as Creon kills Antigone rather than forgive her or admit to the stupidity of his own decree.

Of all the calumnies and condemnations heaped upon Ismene's head, only one is true: like Hegel's slave, she remains attached to life. Only Ismene shows the fluidity and generosity of spirit that refuses to sacrifice relations with real humanbodies to abstract principles or the pride of authority. She never loses her temper with anyone. She is reticent instead of impatient, conciliatory instead of rigid. She is the only one not guilty of sticking fast with heart and head to a rash and intemperate decree. Most important, instead of sticking to the past and the dead, she repeatedly invokes the future. The absolute value for her is living on with those she loves: "What would my life be without you?" Prudent, clever, courageous, absolutely constant, and generous of spirit, Ismene lives on among the living dead who have sacrificed themselves and their sons and daughters to the pride of an abstract principle. Preferring reconciliation to revenge, life to honor, she exhibits the mobility of thought and feeling that makes forgiveness possible.

Perhaps, after all, it is time for feminism and everyone to have done with this oedipal family. Perhaps it is time to remember that it is, after all, *only a play*. So firmly is the story lodged within us, by Hegel and psychoanalysis, as the very template of identity that the narrative has almost come to seem necessary, as if it fell from the sky, from some *topos noetos* where human identity is prefigured.

But it is only a play. And, Hegel's reading of it, in spite of himself, exposes the limits of the fraternal economy and of the rights of Man as the figure of moral life. His reading calls for the deployment of a moral imagination focused on figuring new ways of living on the earth together, for the case of Antigone certainly demonstrates what our own experience only confirms—that our current gender arrangements are not capable of sustaining us.

Antigone dies rather than live with injustice. But we are required constantly to do just that. As Raymond Chandler remarks, "Ours is not a fragrant world."[73] Neither feminist philosophy, which is to say philosophy, nor the future can afford heroines who value the purity of their own conscience or abstract principle over the claims of a living sister.

It is easy to forget that incest, as well as patricide, matricide, fratricide, rape, cannibalism, and other forms of violence and sexual molestation were simply the stuff of Greek culture, at least of its theogony and tragic drama. The story of the brothers' war over property and what is proper to them persists in Anglo-European philosophy as the founding narrative of human community. From Hobbes to Hegel to Freud and Lévi-Strauss, the speculative belief in the violent origin of social relations produces an ethics founded on the rights of Man and a politics founded on the right to property. In this tradition war and social inequity, as well as the subjection of women, are structurally necessary to political community.[74]

Nothing requires that this cruel and violent atmosphere serve as the locus of identity. Nor is there any reason even here to valorize the oedipal story over other stories: the account of a father's willingness to throw his daughter off a cliff in order to put the wind in the sails that will carry him to war (Iphigenia) or the tragic demonstration of how the outrages of fortune can turn even the most noble of women into a raving cur (Hecuba) or the familiar tale of a young wife who, married to an old man, falls in love with her husband's son (Phaedra).[75]

If we cannot have done with this oedipal family, then let us at least not be seduced by Antigone's heroic pose, a mask for her hardheadedness and hardheartedness, into becoming agents of the fraternal economy. Let us stick by Ismene as she takes up the hard work of imagining and securing those infrastructures that would support our life together, that would no longer require that we divide ourselves by the difference of gender, that would prohibit forever the subjection of life to Man's deadly abstractions.

4

Demeter and Persephone, "Unies Sous le Même Manteau"

Mother of loud-shouting, many-shaped Dionysus
Playmate of the beautiful seasons, luminous, of beautiful form,
. . . Your sacred body appears to us in growing fruits and branches. Raped
into your marriage bed in the late autumn
You alone are life and death to distressed mortals,
Persephone. You are forever the nourisher and the death bringer.

—ORPHIC HYMN TO PERSEPHONE

The Eleusinian mysteries must have had a power which the philosophers were unwilling to recognize. It had, above all, a claim to truth, which was recognized by the souls of the *epoptai*. It did not negate the duality of the questing one and the found one. This duality—the scission of the Mother in "mother and daughter"—opened up a vision of the *feminine source of life,* or of the common source of life for men and women alike, just as the sheaf of grain had opened up a vision into the "abyss of the seed." The reason for this is probably that all human beings and not women alone bear this origin and this duality—that *is* both the Mother and the Daughter—within themselves and are therein the heirs of an endless line, not only of fathers but of mothers as well.

—CARL KERÉNYI, ELEUSIS (1991)

THE INSTITUTION OF the rights of man legitimates the privileges of property and (sexual) propriety. The abstraction of these rights abets both the false logic of the generic Man and the fiction of an actual equality.[1] The cultural obsession with the trilogy of the oedipal family reinforces this fraternal logic under which women are both *invisible* in the counsels that determine the future and *hypervisible*, subjected and circulated as the paradigm of property.[2] Under the hegemony of Man and the law of property, women's bodies have always been battlegrounds in the more or less violent disputes among men over property, propriety, and power.

There is no escaping this violent origin, an orgy of rapes, incest, abductions, matricide, cannibalism, and betrayal where virtually every hero comes to a bad end. If we cannot have done with these Greeks, then let us begin again, differently, neither with the fraternal battle over property nor with the dramas of familial desire, but with the only power that ever got the better of Zeus. Thousands of stories circulate across the centuries through hundreds of authors. But here is where it all began.

MOTHERS AND DAUGHTERS: VIOLENCE AND (MATERNAL) POWER

Once upon a time, Demeter strode boldly across the earth, ageless in the opulence of her eternally ripe womanhood. Her great round breasts emitted a fragrant and nourishing atmosphere; the swaying of her wide hips stirred a fertile breeze. As she passed with her vast and elegant gait, the earth responded: perfumes intensified, the loam blackened, the seed sprouted, the bud unfurled.

Unlike her mothers, Rhea and Gaia, who are dispersed throughout the element of the earth, Demeter is gathered into an agency or power. She moves across the earth, and no one acts more decisively than she, not even Zeus.

Rhea and Gaia represent *reactive* powers, subservient to and frustrated by the paternal gods of the revolving sky. Both Gaia and Rhea are defined by an act of revenge against the primal father. Each one undertakes an act of rebellion against an oppressive spouse who refuses to let the children flourish, lest the sons replace him and the daughters be possessed by someone else. Their celestial masters obstruct these maternal terrestrial forces in the very generativity that defines them.

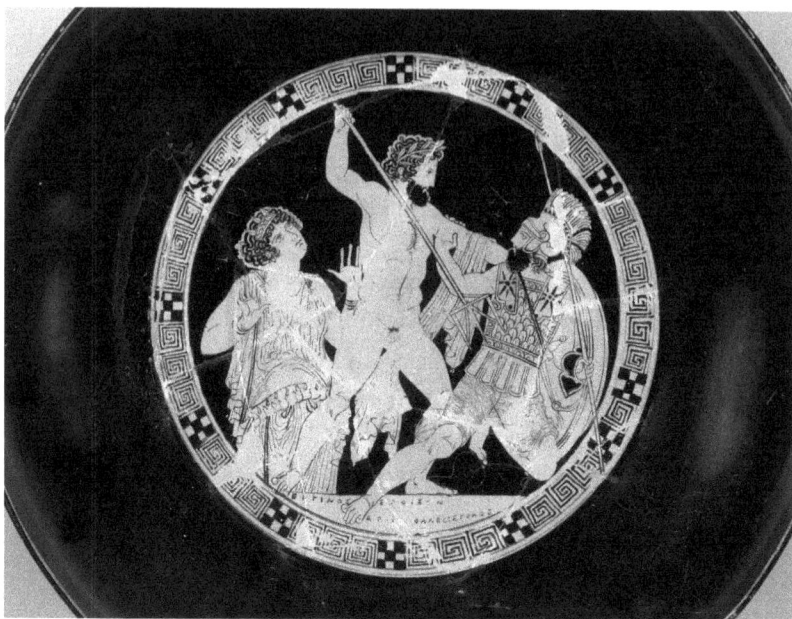

FIGURE. 4.1. Attic red-figured *kylix*, signed by Aristophanes. Antiken Museum Berlin, Beazley Archive 220533

Gaia, half-risen from the earth, submits herself to the lordship of the sky and his brothers, to his surveillance and airpower, the weapons of modern hegemony.[3] Uranus, like a Spartan lord tossing a malformed infant into the pit, forces his children the Cyclopes and Hekatonkheires back into Gaia's womb as they are born. Groaning in pain due to this blockage of her generativity, Gaia challenges her other children the Titans to overthrow their father, and Chronus steps forward to do the deed. Gaia fashions for him an adamantine sickle with terrible jagged teeth. While his brothers hold Uranus down, Chronus castrates their father with the sharp-fanged hook. Uranus' blood rains down upon the ocean, and from the drops emerge the furious Erinnyes as well as the vain and selfish goddess Aphrodite who was destined to cause so much violent trouble for mortals later on.[4]

Chronus, in turn, angers his wife Rhea by eating their children for fear one might supplant him. At the same time, he breaks his alliance with his mother by forcing her children the Cyclopes and Hekatonkheires back into their earthly imprisonment. Counseled by her mother, Rhea substitutes a stone for her youngest son, the infant Zeus, and Chronus swallows the deception. Eventually, with the aid of his mothers and Metis, Zeus drugs his father, administering an emetic that causes Chronus to regurgitate the children he has eaten.[5] These freed siblings, including Demeter, join Zeus in overthrowing Chronus, imprisoning him in the farthest and most desolate reaches of the earth where he had sent his own brothers. Zeus sets the Hekatonkheires to guard their former captor.

Zeus frees the Cyclopes, and, in return, they fashion for him the merciless thunderbolt, as well as the aegis whose shaking creates great storms and deafening thunder. These monstrous brothers invest Zeus with the airpower that ensures his dominion over the gods and the earth. Zeus enjoys unmatched powers of surveillance and bombardment. His arsenal includes missiles, B-52s, and fighter planes, while everyone else is playing with sharp sticks and stones.

While Zeus' form is the airstrike, his powers of surveillance serve not only his physical dominion but also his control of the airwaves or media. No one escapes him. He continually absorbs, recreates, and manufactures intelligence so as to aid his image and interests: lies, boasts, misrepresentations, omissions, elisions, and complete fabrication comprise his regular rhetorical repertoire. As Homer remarks, rumor is Zeus' messenger.[6]

The terrestrial mothers Rhea and Gaia react against the blockage of their generativity, but, as reactive forces, they delegate agency to their children and, above all, to their sons. Ironically, their rebellion against the paternal origin does not release maternal generativity to its own agency; rather, it installs filiation and fraternity as the governing principle. The ascension of Zeus ushers in a new age and dramatically changes the relations among the gods themselves as well as between the gods and mortals. No longer will the relation between father and son be one of threat, violence, and competition. Zeus not only makes an almost perfectly stable peace with his brothers, but he also establishes a maternal, that is nourishing, relation with his sons, who take on the attributes of daughters in caring for their father. The heroes, Zeus' sons by mortal women, are tireless in carrying out his plots and honoring him with their deeds and sacrifices. His divine sons are no less loyal and solicitous in their care for their father and his needs. The chaos and instability of the divine, from the world of the *protogenoi* to the Titans, comes to an end with the victory of Zeus and his brothers. The Olympian generation installs itself as the end of the divine evolution.

From here on, the attention of the gods, though motivated by their own petty jealousies and squabbles, will be fixed almost entirely on the other world of mortal men and women and their affairs. The hierarchies and powers of the gods are settled, and they turn now to the world of men and women as a theater for their lust and glory. With the exception of two brief military interludes, the war with the Giants and the defeat of Typhoës, Zeus spends all his time pursuing immortal or, with greater frequency, mortal beauties and in promoting the welfare of his sons. In their engagement in human affairs, the Olympians are themselves articulated. The gods no longer appear as elements or natural powers, but differentiate themselves as individualized agencies with specific historical effects.

Zeus produces the age of the heroes, in which the wars of mortals are fought, not by fathers and sons but between brothers and their tribes. Men, the heroes, the brothers, fight for the three reasons Hobbes identifies as essential both to the citizen and to the state: security, property, and glory. In rare cases—Hektor, for example, and possibly Odysseus, whose reluctance to leave Ithaca for Troy is legendary—heroes fight defensively, reluctantly, to secure their domains from attack. More often, they fight, as Hobbes remarks, for "gain," using "violence, to make themselves Masters of other men's persons, wives, children, and cattell."[7] While the right to property is instituted to secure privilege and justify social inequity, the logic of brotherhood always breeds tribalism, violence, and war. Filiation and fraternity have always set severe practical limits on the abstract idea of universal freedom and opportunity. In fraternal regimes, disciplinary force regulates the institutions and boundaries of citizenship, while vast military infrastructures remain poised to extend or defend the *domaine* against other tribes. The Greeks fought over women and land no less than men do today. Mortals still live in the age of the heroes, where fraternal orders do battle over property and power. While the twentieth century was defined by the tribal war between France and Germany, the twenty-first century seems poised to be defined by the tribal war between Sunni and Shia. American politics in the twenty-first century also exhibits features of tribal warfare in which the defeat of the opposing side is more important than public policy and welfare. Tribalism, as Hegel warned, always prevents the emergence of those corporate public agencies and collaborations that are necessary to address pervasive social problems undermining the welfare of the community.[8]

As for the force of "glory" in mortal affairs, it remains significant globally as well, whether as religious fanaticism, "patriotism," "nationalism," "honor," or "face." Men interpreting religious law required that Mukhtaran Mai be raped to restore to other men their (family's) honor. Military recruiters and politicians regularly deploy appeals to national pride to convince young mortals that there is something magnificent in risking their lives on behalf of the ruling powers. Every state, whether religious or not, promises some kind of glory, from a Main Street parade to eternal life, to those who are convinced to die for it. States refuse to desist from pursuing nuclear weapons or indulge in displays of force as a matter of national honor. Like Antigone and Hegel's master, the heroes risk life in order to prove their virtue superior to it: this is their glory. They elevate the law of their heart above the living presence of one human being to another, putting at risk generativity itself.

Still, no one could claim to testify with more authority on the matter of glory in human affairs than great Achilles of the swift feet, the most glorious warrior of all. When Odysseus encounters his spirit in the underworld, Achilles greets him with lamentation and alarm: "How could you endure to come down here to Hades' place, where the senseless dead men dwell, mere imitations of perished mortals?"[9] Odysseus responds by reminding Achilles of his glorious renown among the living and the authority of his glory among the dead. Achilles counters that he cannot be consoled for dying: "I would rather be a humble farmer on earth, than the greatest hero among the dead."[10]

◆　◆　◆　◆

Under the hegemony of Zeus and his brothers, Demeter's share in the Olympians' original division of dominion is often forgotten, strategically erased in the telling and retelling of these tales. Poseidon takes possession of the sea and its creatures, Hades is installed as king of the dead, and Zeus reigns supreme as the master of airpower, but the earth in its generativity is assigned to Demeter.

Rhea and Gaia remain fixed in stone, fixed in the ancient body of the earth as a pervasive and generalized generativity of the earth. The earth embodies the difference between this fixed, steadfast being of stone and the profusion of living things. Stone accrues time. It awaits the engraving force and the pull of gravity and offers itself up to the arc of the sky.

Demeter, however, does not live under or in the earth, even though she engenders the fecundity of the soil, nor does she raise her arms in submission to any celestial power.[11] Unlike the reactive power of her mothers, Demeter's generative power is gathered into an agency that nurtures, tends, and facilitates living things. Under her mantle, everything is more flavorful, refreshing, and nourishing. She frequently appears at wells, imparting to the water the fresh cold clarity of a pristine mountain spring, and she never misses a chance to nurse a promising infant.

Long before the business with Persephone is resolved and the struggle of life and death that had threatened everything, domesticated in a stable motion, long before she lost herself in the search for her daughter, Demeter takes her place at the wedding celebration of Cadmus and Harmony.[12] The union inaugurates a new era of domesticity in the relations of gods and humans and foreshadows the god who will walk among men, almost as if he were one of them. At the nuptial feast, the beauty of the farmer Iasion excites Demeter's open, generous heart, and she lies with him there and then in the fertile ground of a newly plowed field.[13] This hasty amorous encounter on the earth testifies to the goddess' confident sovereignty in her own sexuality and to her love of the sensuous realm, as well as to the reciprocity of the couple's affections. In the mutuality of their desire, she and Iasion enact a relation among gods and mortals that figures a new sexuality and the possibility of new forms of life among mortals.

When Demeter sees a handsome farmer at a wedding, she does not hesitate to indulge her desire. She enjoys a long life of mutual pleasure and growth with her callipygian husband and their children. Invoking neither the violent lust of Zeus nor the uxorious revenge of her mothers and her sisters, Demeter answers to and speaks of the needs and pleasures of every humanbody in relation to the element of the earth. Against the sexual violence and hysteria of the oedipal narrative, Demeter figures a sexuality that is unabashedly *agricultural*: Demeter cultivates Iasion and is cultivated by him in every register. They confidently enjoy the sexuality of their bodies, just as they frankly savor the sensuous pleasures of the earth, of food and drink. Their candid relationship cultivates the nature of each and proves generative beyond their own issue.

Iasion and Demeter collaborate in the generative projects of farming, teaching the farming both of crops and of animals. Iasion is sometimes described as a hunter rather than a farmer, but the contradiction is easily resolved. Iasion's skill in hunting is not in killing but in capturing live animals and domesticating them. This mortal herdsman and his animal husbandry foreshadow Demeter's grandson Dionysus who is also known for his skill in capturing and domesticating animals. At the time of Cadmus wedding, Demeter has not yet given mortals the knowledge of how to cultivate the earth that will produce fixed settlements and complex civilizations. The quasi-nomadic practices of the herder mediated between the itinerant hunter-gatherer and the localized community of the farmer. While the farmer remains in place, and the hunter-gatherer may wander indefinitely, the herder travels with the weather, but on a regular itinerary, according to a logic of return. Far from aimless, herders are nevertheless always between places. Herders, who farm animals instead of crops, represent the moment of transition when mortals cease to be simply animals that must eat and become animals for whom eating is an ethical and political act.[14]

Many authors repeat Zeus' boast that, at the wedding of Cadmus and Harmony, he struck Iasion dead on the spot for his impertinence in lying with the goddess. Zeus' bluster amounts to no more than a feeble attempt to reassert his own property rights; nevertheless, his lie takes hold, in spite of the goddess' own testimony that she married Iasion. Ever modest in the prodigious amplitude of her generosity, Demeter lived with this handsome farmer and loved him into his old age.[15] They had several sons, and, given Demeter's love of fertile soil and her propensity for simple living, it is likely that she spent most of her time on his farm.

Demeter tends both the elements of life on Earth—air, fire, earth, and water—and living beings themselves. As she strides across the earth, the apparently endless cycle of the seasons turns and returns. Fall and winter will become spring and summer again. Life first appears in this becoming of the seasons or the elements of life: dry seasons and rainy seasons, midnight suns and full moons. Demeter guards and, in her motion, sustains the reassuringly regular rhythms of this elemental vitality.

At the same time, Demeter shelters all things that grow, all creatures that are not stone. Life, as becoming, manifests itself not only in the circular motion of the elements but also in the linear birth and growth of living beings, plants, and animals. Within this sheltering, Demeter attends differently to human mortals than to all other animals. The destiny of other animals is determined by the *differentiae*: beak and talon or tooth and claw. The destiny of the eagle or the lion is inscribed in its very body. It makes no sense to hold the eagle responsible for eating the rabbit or the lion for eating the antelope, but the plasticity of the human brain, hand, and foot leaves destiny undetermined and in question. Living human beings are constantly answering this question, telling certain stories, holding hands or a sword, looking backward at guilt and debt or forward to the future.

Demeter's interest in the embodied freedom of mortals takes the form of a pedagogical agency. As she strides across the earth, Demeter brings the fertile seed. The seed is an abyss: it embodies an infinite legacy of generation and generativity.[16] The seed teaches the necessity of respect for living things, for it will not sprout if mistreated. The seed teaches the necessity of respect for what we eat, what sacrifices itself, animal and plant, for our nourishment. The seed teaches the necessity of imagining the future and acting for the future, as not everything grown can be eaten. Some seed must be saved for the next planting. The seed teaches us to act on behalf of the generation that will come after us.

Demeter also brings the articulated technology of agriculture and water that will transform wanderers into people of place. Demeter teaches mortals the practices and strategies necessary to cultivate Earth as a sustaining home. All the Olympians take an eager interest in the affairs of mortals, but their interventions almost invariably involve sexual conquest or a spirit of revenge. Demeter is rare, if not unique, among the gods in acting disinterestedly, out of a love for things that grow and an active interest in promoting the generativity of the earth and in improving the life of mortals. Demeter and her grandson actively cultivate the earth by teaching men and women what and how to eat.

Demeter's motivation lies neither in the desire to possess nor in *ressentiment*. Her spring is joy. More than any other god or goddess, Demeter enjoys her access to the sensuous dimensions of the mortal human body. She eats with relish and enjoys with abandon the lithe, brown body of her beautiful husband. Even as she wanders, dejected and heartsick, searching for her daughter, she cannot help but enjoy a frieze of young girls. Befriending them at the well near Eleusis in the realm of Celeus, she cannot help but offer to nurture their little brother, with whom she attempts to share all her radiant gifts.[17] Despite her despair,

Demeter cannot help but laugh from her belly at the bawdy, ribald jokes of the old Iambe. Joy in the sensuous bodies of living things and a constant generativity define her agency.

Demeter is as different from her sisters, particularly Hera, as she is from her mothers. Hera, like their mother and grandmother, exerts only a reactive force, constantly raging against Zeus' infidelities and seeking revenge for them. Though Demeter enjoys a long, fruitful, and happy marriage to Iasion, she is not defined by it. She never exhibits any jealousy, nor does she have any reason to do so.

Demeter takes no part in the petty quarrels and jealousies or the vicious pride of her sisters. Her laughter marks a joyous responsiveness to the sensuous surprises of Earth, but her stories contain no evidence of vanity or vainglory. She intervenes in mortal affairs only out of a love for the pleasures of the flesh and a generative relation to human animals, as a generous agent of instruction and metamorphosis. She is a servant of life, of becoming, both the cyclical life of the elements and the birth and growth of living beings.[18]

It is true that, in the end, Demeter's wrath proves far more terrible than the jealous rages of Hera, her power far greater than Hera's strategies of revenge, but it arises only on behalf of another, her daughter, who was raped and taken away in the hour of her shining spring.

LIFE / DEATH:
SHADOW OF THE FROLICKING GIRLS

Before Demeter's marriage to Iasion, long before the abduction of the maiden, there had already been violence, for the maiden herself is the result of an incestuous rape.[19] Though Demeter is no more able to defend herself against her brother's attack than any of his other divine and human victims, she responds generously with the most refreshing and beautiful of creatures, the girl Kore, who was, from the beginning, like the return of spring. The maiden radiated with the commencement of life: life that is still growing into itself, that is not yet itself, but promises itself with an irresistible luminosity and joy that engages every eye and heart. Like the green of spring, fairer and fresher than all the rest, Kore glows with the future and possibility.

Of all the metaphysical twaddle that is heaped upon the girl's head, nothing could be more antithetical to her nature than the claim that she is a unique being or origin, hidden beyond life, to be pursued interminably by male gods and philosophers. Kore belongs always to *a frieze of blooming young girls*.[20] She exists as a member of an ensemble of daughters.

> *We were all in the beautiful meadow—*
> *Leukippê; Phaino; Elektra; and Ianthê;*
> *Melitê; Iachê; Rhodeia; and Kallirhoê;*
> *Melibosis; Tychê; and flower-faced Okyrhoê;*
> *Khryseis; Ianeira; Akastê; Admetê;*
> *Rhodopê; Plouto, and lovely Kalypso;*
> *Styx; Ourania; and fair Galaxaura; Pallas,*
> *rouser of battles; and Artemis, sender of arrows—*
> *playing and picking lovely flowers with our hands,*
> *soft crocus mixed with irises and hyacinth,*
> *rosebuds and lilies, a marvel to see, and the*
> *narcissus that wide earth bore like a crocus.*[21]

The Oceanides with whom Kore plays in the beautiful meadow embody the colors and motion of clouds, a chiasm of air, water, and fire, as well as the fluid forms of water. Together, they comprise the elements—air, fire, water, earth— of life on Earth. Together, they make up the phases of the day for all living creatures: now Rhodeia and Rhodopê in the rose gold of early morning, then Khryseis in the yellow light of noon, and finally Ianthê and Elektra in the violet and amber hues of sunset. Together, they generate the refreshing fluidity and vital motion of fresh water in all its forms: Kallirhoê's downpours and effusive springs, Leukippê's frothy streams, Plouto's fertile rains, Admetê's storms, Galaxaura's mists, and Okyrhoê's swift creeks and rills. Melitê guards the sweetness and purity of water, while Iachê celebrates the joy of water to a thirsty being or to a thirsty land. These shining young girls shelter the passing of the day and the nourishing mobility of water as the fundamental conditions of life on earth. Becoming, life, exists at the intersection of the elements and the phases of the day.[22]

The girls also shelter the knowledge and labor that cultivate the earth to sustain living beings. Plouto embodies not only the fecundity of water but also its receptivity to human management for human ends. She anticipates the agricultural knowledge that Demeter and Dionysus will give to mortals, just as Iachê anticipates the ecstasies of the Eleusinian mysteries on which she will attend. Melibosis evokes green pastures and fruit trees in reminder of the dependence of all food on the vitality of water and in honor of the collaboration between humans and other animals. Playing quietly among the other girls, Kalypso reminds us that water often likes to hide itself, while Styx will not allow us to forget the horror of poisoned water, nor Tychê the fragility of life itself.

Kore, the maiden, belongs to this tribe of girls as the unity of all its aspects. She looks back to comprise and reflect, a look in which all the radiations of life are complicated, the I / eye in which the dimensions and perspectives of life participate. Kore belongs to the ensemble as the part / member reflecting the whole by *looking back*.[23] Everything vital is implicated in her as the spring of life: *Omnia complicans.* Perhaps, the Oceanides attend the goddess; perhaps the virginal goddesses attend their half-sister Kore. Who can say? In any case, Kore echoes Iachê's cry of joy. She reflects all the girls, the thrill of refreshment in all its forms, the fertility of well-watered ground, the hues of the changing sky, and the metamorphic mobility of water, but also the hidden spring, the poisoned stream, and the inevitability of death.

Many readers, Calasso and Derrida among them, assume that Kore sees herself reflected for the first time in the eye of her abductor.[24] Kore, however, has eyes only for her band of girls. It is in them that she discovers herself, and it is the vitality of this band that she displays. Her truth is not the eye of Hades but the frieze of blooming young girls with whom she celebrates life's efflorescence. Her agency is not yet mediated by death, but only by the surge and joy and unpredictable variety of life and its conditions. She is susceptible to the surveillance of Zeus, but Kore's own ocular power belongs to the other girls and the natural powers they shelter: the frieze of girls, becoming, life itself, the return of spring.

Because she is taken just as she bends to pick a narcissus, some authors blame Kore for her own abduction, as if the identity of the flower were in itself a condemnation of some deadly self-absorption on her part.[25] In these stories she has, through vanity or some other base desire, allowed her eye to be attached by the wrong thing. This mean misinterpretation undermines the girl's agency as well as the solidarity of the band of girls, and it ignores altogether the relevant Boeotian beliefs about Narcissus. It was in Boeotia on the plain of Nysa that Persephone was raped and Dionysus born for the first time. According to Pausanius, the Boeotians believe that Narcissus was mourning his beloved twin sister.[26] His reflection in the spring gives him the soothing illusion that she is still there *before his own eyes looking back,* a living presence. A living being stands before the loving eye in its caressing gaze, two members of the same vital presence.

The narcissus represents not the narcissism of psychoanalysis but the impossible mourning of a brother for his irredeemably lost sister. The depth of his love measures her absence, the depth of his loss. His suffering marks the difference between the living presence of the sister and the impossible presence of the dead sister who nevertheless lives on in him. The depth of his suffering measures the degree to which he was her, his relation to her, the degree to which she animated him.

As the inverse of Antigone's glorious death, Narcissus pines away beside the spring, fading into the lush moss and stones, and Gaia turns the beauty of his sorrow into the lovely redolent flower, almost as early and profuse in its bloom as the carpets of dainty lavender crocus. These tall, dazzling, yellow blooms trumpet spring and are as quickly gone, like the surge of love in the living who die.

Other authors reflect more of Zeus' rumormongering and implicate Gaia in the rape: she is said to have created the irresistible flower, at the command of Zeus, precisely for the purpose of ensnaring the eye of the maiden. The flower itself testifies otherwise. The intense profusion of its perfume evokes the deep green of the forest floor, wet stones, and the earthy sweetness of rich black soil teeming with life. Its joyous, jaunty invocation of spring belongs to the mothers and their girls. Gaia created it to please the girls as a floral tribute to their shining spring. Typically, Zeus works to obscure the agency of the mothers, claiming it as his own, and his authors try ceaselessly to undermine the solidarity of mothers and daughters.[27]

Demeter will not give up her search until her daughter is once again *before her own eyes.*[28] She will not allow her daughter to be taken from her. She will take no one's word; nothing will substitute for the living presence of the daughter herself. She will have nothing less than her daughter *before her own eyes looking back.*

The well-worn tale of Persephone's abduction by Hades provides cover for what really happened, just as the story of Semele masks the real birth of Dionysus. It was Zeus who first spied the luminous maiden cavorting with her companions in a meadow of flowers. So great was his lust, Nonnus observes, that *his eyes ran ahead of him* and could not get enough of her.[29] After dancing with her maidens on a hot day, Kore loosened her *gurdle* and unfastened her brooches, letting her *chiton* fall to the soft, mossy bank of a cool stream. While she bathed, Zeus ravaged her breast with his eyes, driven mad by his lascivious appetite. She cannot escape his eye. It was he who came among the girls and took her virginity forever, leaving her pregnant with the god of wine and theater.

Almost immediately, he realizes the gravity of what he has done. While he certainly wishes to avoid the troublesome wrath of his infinitely and eternally jealous wife, it is Demeter who suddenly strikes him with a fear he has never known. Everything else Zeus does follows from the double intention to hide the child from Hera and to hide the mother from her own mother.

When she discovers that Kore, the maiden, has disappeared from the meadows of her shining spring, Demeter wanders the earth in search of her daughter, her mournful cries unceasing. Most of the stories offer this figure of Demeter, as if she were forever the bereft mother carrying aloft two great flaming torches as she searches far and wide for her missing child. But this was only the beginning.

Zeus conspires with his brothers to prevent Demeter from discovering the rape. Poseidon, ever quarrelsome and bullish, resented Demeter's dominion over the earth and wished to see her suffer, while his elder brother Hades had dared to desire the girl himself. Zeus distracts Demeter with the Tantalus affair, where her generativity is again required to save Pelops; and Poseidon assaults her while she rests among the herds of Apollo in the form of a horse.[30] Only after the delay imposed by these detours and assaults does Demeter arrive at Eleusis, where, with the help of Hecate, she discovers the truth.

Meanwhile, Zeus has arranged with Hades to sequester the maiden in the realm of the dead. Just this once, the god of the dead will be allowed to transgress the border of the living and carry off the maiden whose cheeks still bloom.[31] What greater revenge might Hades exact for his lot among the dead, where there is no taste and everything is a bloodless shadow of itself, than to subdue life in its budding beauty, at the very moment of its efflorescence, as yet unspoiled by any use or desire. He does not know until he carries her off what change has already been wrought in her by his brother.

For the younger brother, Zeus himself, whom fate favored with the supremacy of airpower: what better place to hide Kore after the rape than among the dead, where her mother will never think to look for her living daughter, where indeed Demeter, as life itself, cannot go. Women are always being abducted in these tales; however, this abduction is unique: this is *the* abduction, when the generative power of the mother and the joyful girlhood of the daughter are made subject to the brothers' violent logic of property and war. Kore becomes Persephone, the "one who brings destruction," and can never again be the girl blooming among the flowers.

What violence takes place between the daughter and the father few narrators have dared to say. The cover story—Hera's jealousy, Semele's vanity, the implantation of the unformed Dionysus in Zeus' thigh—successfully obscured what really happened. It is unlikely, as some authors report, that he came to Kore in the guise of a snake or dragon, her mother's animals. Had he been so close to the ground in his approach, Demeter would have detected him. Because Zeus took the maiden from Nysa to Crete, at least one author suggests that he came to her in the shape of a bull, as he had to Europa, playing with the other girls among the flowers.[32] Certainly, it is not hard to imagine the beautiful, fragrant white bull coming among the girls in the meadow, just as it had approached Europa and her companions from the sea. This author argues that Zeus brought Persephone to Crete in order to borrow Pasiphae's apparatus.[33]

In fact, the tale of Semele's immolation was a confused appropriation of what really happened, promoted by Zeus himself to keep both Hera and Demeter off the track. To Kore, the maiden herself, Zeus came as the bolt of lightning. Not for her an animal, however magnificent, nor anything so mundane as a shower of gold. Just this once, with this impossibly beautiful incarnation of the urgency and freshness of young life, Zeus was himself in all his airpower and glory.

The maiden was no mortal, and there was no reason at all for her to have any commerce with the dead or their ruler. Kore is the freshness of the air, the rich loamy scent of an earth suffused with life. Her fragrant atmosphere replenishes and nourishes the spirit as the intense scent of an opening rose dilates the nose and infuses the body with its perfume. She might have remained suspended at the beginning of life like the sparkle of dew outlining the burgeoning leaves on a day, bright and cool, in early spring. But it was not to be.

When Zeus penetrated her, he split her in two, as lightning does the tree. He created a shadow or memory that could no longer be absorbed in her presence, a loss that could not be undone. She became the life that dies while the other lives on. Marked forever and everywhere from here on by the difference between mother and daughter, life became sustainable only as death and regeneration. So Kore, who with her mother comprised the principle of life, became Persephone, the principle of life / death, of the destruction that is essential to life. While Demeter shelters the vital elements and the becoming of generations, as well as the birth and growth of all living things, Persephone shelters mortals in the logic of life / death. Persephone, "the one who brings destruction," only does so in the service of life and the future. Beyond the opposition between life and death that defined the difference between mortal and immortal, Persephone embodies the immanence of death in life. As Rilke remarks, "The living make too great a distinction between the living and the dead."[34] Life depends, as Hegel and Proust demonstrate, on many deaths of many selves.[35] As principle of generation and life, Persephone is also the "death bringer." The girl who is born of a mother will become a mother herself: generations age and die, yielding the future to those who come after. This double identity of mother / daughter constitutes Persephone and all mortals: she is at once the daughter of Demeter, mother of Dionysus, and the Queen of the Dead. Every mortal is born of a woman. Every mortal will give way to the generations that come after. Every mortal exists in the realm of the living *and the dead.*

COLLABORATING AGENCIES: CONSTANCY, GENERATIVITY, SOLIDARITY

At Eleusis Demeter finally discovered what had happened to her daughter.

Through the aid of Hecate and sustained by the hospitality of the house of King Celeus, Demeter discovers that Hades has transgressed the borders of the living and the dead at Eleusis, crossing over to steal her daughter from among the flowers. Some say she consulted Helios and forced him to admit that he had seen Hades abduct her daughter while Zeus looked on, but Demeter hardly needed his testimony to know that Hades would never have dared this scandalous incursion into the body of the living earth without the connivance of his brother, whose power of surveillance was absolute and unrelenting.

Demeter does not even give Zeus the courtesy of an audience. She makes no appeal and will hear none. She merely withdraws her power from the earth so that nothing grows. Buds shrivel, seeds fail to sprout, the vine withers, and the earth grows cold and hard. Zeus attempts to negotiate, but Demeter will have nothing less than her living daughter back among the living. Only her daughter, here and now, *before her own eyes looking back* will suffice.[36]

Zeus is lord of all things: his brothers bend to his will, but he cannot command the refreshing mobility of fresh water or the fecundity of the earth without which the warm, quivering flesh of life crumbles to dust and ashes. The utter barrenness of the earth compels Zeus to relent and to renege on his contract with his brother Hades. He yields to Demeter because he must: without her, there is no life, and without the drama of human life, the gods will neither smell the smoke of sacrifice nor have any theater for their lust and glory.

Here, hidden in the heart of all these tales where sons are regularly abandoned by fathers who fear being supplanted and fathers are regularly killed by sons who erect a new fraternal order, is the story of a mother who, in spite of the odds and against the greatest of powers, will not give up her daughter. Her maternal fidelity proves decisive. For Zeus she is *the* woman, the only power that ever gets the better of him.

Zeus' penetration of his sister, of the fecundity of women and the earth, yields the luminous maiden, but it also produces the figure of a new social unit, the mother and daughter "wrapped in the same cloak."[37] The daughter is herself already a mother. Persephone and Demeter represent the difference of mother and daughter as a difference articulated within each and all, within every humanbody. The difference is not only a figure of solidarity but also a difference internal to each one who will be supplanted by those who come after in the generativity of life / death.

They sit quietly off to the side in salle 36, vitrine 25. Somewhere in that endless series of rooms in the Louvre that houses Greek, Roman, and Etruscan antiquities, somewhere between the cold, generic mothers of the Cyclades, all angles and stylized curves, and the specific personalities of the Hellenes, they sit quietly "unies sous le même mânteau." This small, obscure terra cotta figurine

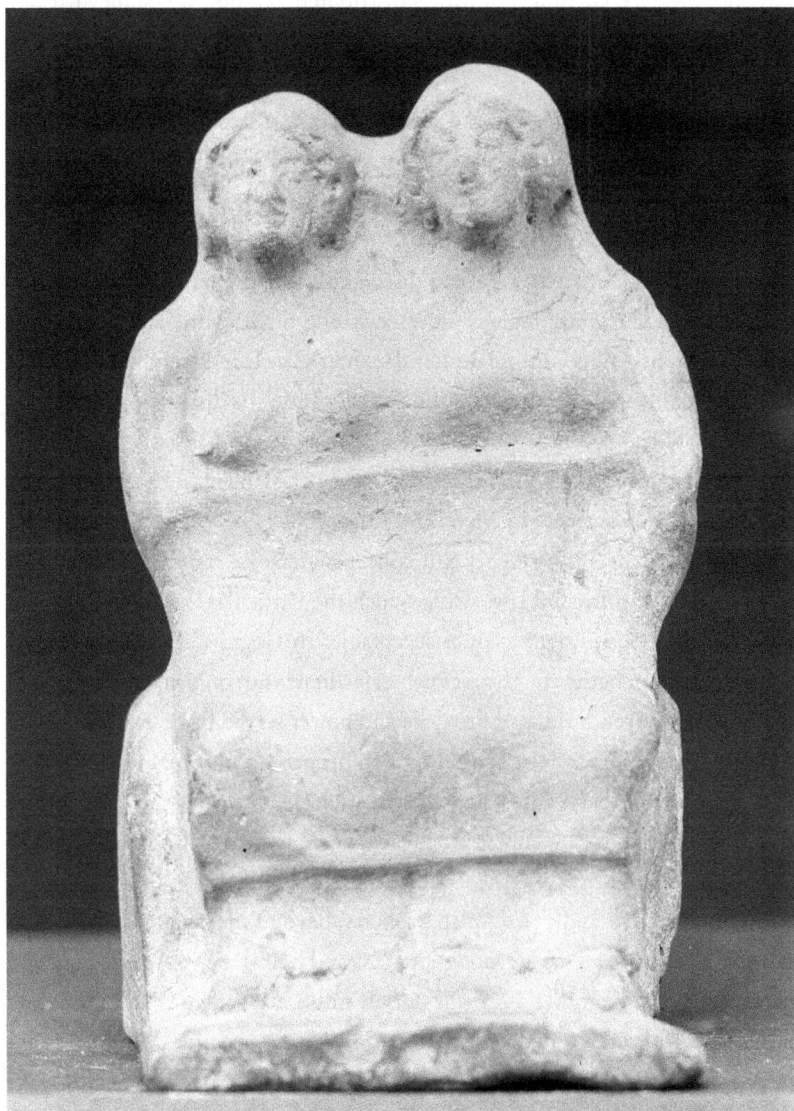

FIGURE. 4.2. Double divinity, h. 8.9 cm, Greek, ca. 450, from Cyzique[?].
Copyright © Musée du Louvre, dist. RMN-Grand Palais / Art Resource, NY

was once produced in bulk and widely distributed, but now it is somewhat rare and hard to find. In all the vast collection of the Louvre, only here do they sit "unies sous le même mânteau."[38] Two heads, side by side, happy and robust; four breasts aligned in a row above the shelf of their two crossed arms; four knees, imperfectly aligned, as Persephone's right knee breaks slightly to the right. The firm taught thighs of both are visible beneath their drapery. They have walked far before this moment of rest; four feet, and again Persephone's right foot angles slightly to the right. One can distinguish the mother from the mother-daughter by the slightly higher, more enclosing pitch of the shoulder as she reaches with her other arm across her daughter's back: indissoluble, sustaining one another in a perfect pitch of stillness that cannot be disturbed. Constancy. Intimacy. Solidarity.

Zeus produces the hero and the great history of Man's mastery of nature and the mastery of the nature in Man. The great work of reproducing nature and ordinary experience in thoughts and concepts creates a realm of invisibilities, a dimension of forms and laws, from which the particular is rendered only an instance and its loss insignificant or acceptable. This logic of the generic, the reduction of difference in the abstract name, facilitates not only normalizing force but also the concentrations of privilege and power served by it. The rhetoric of rights will always have been complicit with property and sexual propriety and with the violence that secures them. Declarations of abstract rights may sanitize certain regimes, but they substitute for real urgency in actually engaging social inequities and injustices and the violence that sustains them.

Beyond the law and the right to property, beyond the rational calculations of debts and entitlements, beyond judgment and punishment, there is *the claim of the right* in the mother who will not abandon her daughter and the moral imperative of the mother / daughter who impose a logic of life / death that is not built around violence and the dispute over property or sexual propriety. Unlike Antigone's claim, Demeter's does not honor the dead brother, but demands the living daughter *before her own eyes looking back*.

While Demeter shelters elemental vitality and the cycle of seasons, as well as the generativity of animals and plants, Persephone shelters the becoming / mortality of humanbodies and all life. She embodies life / death, the death in life, life as many deaths, death as essential to life. She brings into the midst of the gods the logic of life and death that afflicts all Earth's creatures. The regeneration that is essential to life, which is reflected in the cyclical time of earth, requires for individual creatures a linear temporality of growth, birth, and death. The time of mortals and all living creatures is not cyclical and does not return, but comes to an end just as abrupt as its beginning. Demeter shelters living on Earth; Persephone shelters living and dying on Earth.

Like her mother, and in contrast to the other gods, Persephone's intercession with human beings has nothing to do with sex or war. For the few human beings who transgress the boundary between life and death, Persephone proves a generous and faithful ally. She allows Orpheus to rescue Eurydice, because she is moved by his song. She returns Alcestis to the living in recognition of her heroism. She welcomes Herakles like the brother that he is and does all she can to assist him in his labors.

Persephone brings destruction in the service of generation and generativity. She embodies the logic of life / death at the heart of life itself in the individual, in the species, and in Earth. Life is not the opposite of death, but shot through with many deaths, many metamorphoses in which something dies so that something else may live. The boy dies in the man and will not return. The son is not the reincarnation of the father, but a new *coup de dés*, a new and unique life. The girl among the flowers, who "was raped into her marriage bed," becomes the mother / daughter.[39] The linearity and finitude of the individual creature's life intersects the no less finite cycle of Earth's regeneration in the I / eye of Persephone who embodies the unique loss incurred in each individual death.

This double difference between life and death, between the mother and the daughter, installs a logic of intergenerational generativity even as it marks the irreparable loss of each irreducible humanbody.[40] The curious *aporia* of the now—the permanent form of an evaporating content that is, nonetheless, *what is*—marks the species and life itself no less than the specific humanbody.[41] As generativity, life—the life of living bodies in their element—necessarily implies that the body continually supplants itself, that it lives as "many deaths of many selves" and that it will be supplanted by those who come after. Life, generativity, embodies an intergenerational logic of life / death on which both the identity of the specific humanbody and the claims of ethics depend. Demeter and Persephone wrapped in the same cloak: a collaborative agency that is neither configured in relations of care and dependency nor in economic exchanges of debt and entitlement, judgment and punishment. Demeter will not abandon her daughter, and not even Zeus can defeat her. Persephone accepts the necessity of her role as the living queen of the realm of the dead in order to embody among the living the ethics of life / death.[42] Together, she and her mother embody the chiasm of Earth and the individual, the cycle of seasons and the mortality of each creature. However this collaboration may have been obscured, it is this intersection of the cyclical regeneration of the seasons with the linear temporality of the finite animal that makes possible both the generativity of nature and the tides of generation that sustain human life.

Persephone never appears alone. She is always with her mother, who cannot cross into the land of the dead, or always with her husband, who cannot again cross into the land of the living except to collect the wounded from the battlefield. Persephone exists always with each one across an impossible border. It would be absurd to think that the Queen of Death might not be there to welcome her guests when they arrived.[43]

Yet, she is always with her mother.

Persephone draws her cloak around her; she leans in to whisper to her mother. Demeter supports her turgid breast, ever ready to nurse. Demeter will have nothing less than her daughter before her own eyes looking back. She will be animated again by her daughter's living presence and nothing else. What looks back at us commands respect: *re-spectus*, looking back. Demeter is never alone either: her daughter is always there looking back.

Demeter and Persephone do figure nature as feminine and the feminine body as continuous with nature. To embrace them as ethical figures requires recognition of this continuity of the human body with the natural and elemental world on which it depends.[44] The life of living beings depends on the life-sustaining elements of air, water, earth, and fire. In our time, Irigaray argues, science and technological "progress," in complicity with capital, have put the elemental itself in danger.[45] Earth and its elements provide the element of life for humanbodies. Sustaining humanbodies, Earth also lays on them the claim of the right. Rather than Man imposing a relation of mastery on nature and on his own nature, nature imposes on men and women the responsibility to look back at their

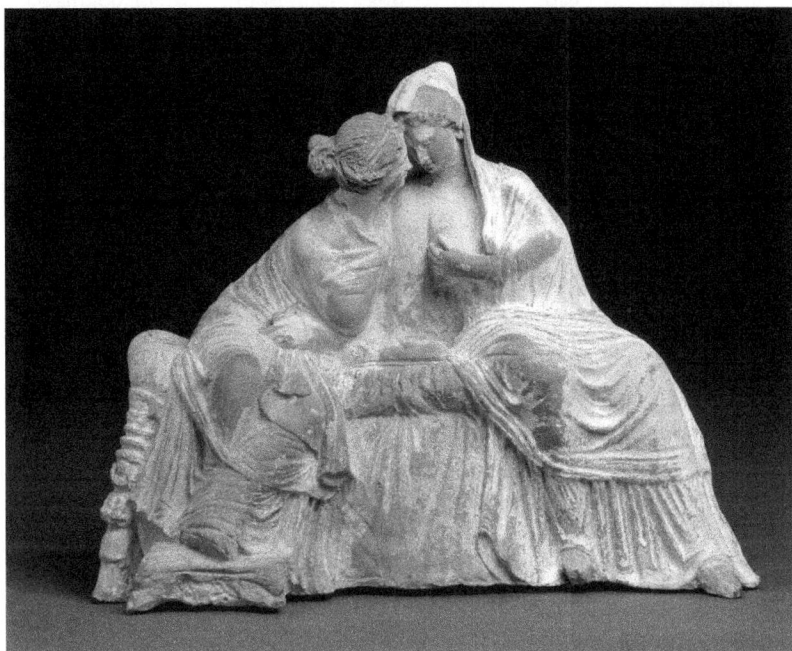

FIGURE 4.3. Terra-cotta group of two female figures (perhaps Demeter and Persephone), h. 20.5 cm, l. 25.4 cm, Hellenistic, ca. 100 BC. Myrina [?]. Copyright © The Trustees of the British Museum

dependency on nature and on the generativity and generosity of other living beings, plants and animals. Hobbes figured nature in the twin tits of land and sea from which Man sucks life.[46] Demeter and Persephone refigure nature and humans in nature in relations of intergenerational generativity. They impose on men and women the claim of the right, not a debt to be paid or a privilege to be owned, but a future to be served.

An ethics of life serves the elemental conditions of life and the wild profusion of differentiated beings, as well as the continuities and collaboration between humanbodies and other animals, each one commanding respect, a looking back at the interdependencies and integrities that bind and distinguish all living beings. The distance and universality of words that sustained the project of abstraction and the generic Man here give rise to respect or looking back. What is most particular, my-death, is yet something absolutely universal; in looking back at the others who have sustained life, the creature of words and signs answers to the claim of the right and intergenerational generativity.

Persephone supplements her mother's regenerative powers with the necessity of death to life. Together they collaborate to nourish and promote the welfare of mortals, teaching them how to cultivate a field and safeguard the vital mobility of water. The culture of farming introduced a new attachment to place and respect for the specificity of landscape and climate. Agriculture brings respect for what nourishes and the labor that cultivates it. Demeter and her children taught men and women the techniques of a way of life that respects the element of the earth while enjoying its generosity. Their agriculture and viniculture combine the most intense and satisfying sensuality with the most rigorous of disciplines. These activities supply basic needs, but they also form agency. Farming requires imagination, a respect for the future, and deferred desire. It is in agriculture that humans first learned to delay gratification. Women, tied to a place by child rearing, gathered seeds but did not eat them all. Some were saved and returned to the earth, and this gratitude was met with yet more generosity in the form of the new plant. Ten thousand years ago, women and men followed the two mothers in tilling and planting, managing water and herding sheep, feeding themselves, forming themselves, forming associations by learning how to cultivate nature together.

Blinded by the screen of the oedipal triangle, inserting itself as the lens of identity, readers may have forgotten the other stories where generativity repairs violence, generosity welcomes the uncertainty of the new, and solidarity binds mothers together across generations.

PART THREE
Livable Futures

The important thing really, I feel, is to know what is to be done and how to do what is necessary to guarantee the existence of a world that is livable in the future, livable in a way that, hopefully, is more human, happier, that is less prey to the instinct to dominate and to possess the other, above all the other sex, the other gender.

—LUCE IRIGARAY, *DEMOCRACY BEGINS BETWEEN TWO* (1994)

The movement by which, not without effort and uncertainty, dreams and illusions, one detaches oneself from what is accepted as true and seeks other rules—that is philosophy. The displacement and transformation of frameworks of thinking, the changing of received values and all the work that has been done to think otherwise, to do something else, to become other than what one is—that too is philosophy.

—MICHEL FOUCAULT, "THE MASKED PHILOSOPHER" (1980)

Recovering the feminine principle as respect for life in nature and society appears to be the only way forward for men as well as women, in the North as well as the South. The metaphors and concepts of minds deprived of the feminine principle have been based on seeing nature and women as worthless and passive, and finally as dispensable. These ethnocentric categorisations have been universalized, and with their universalisation has been associated the destruction of nature and the subjugation of women. But this dominant mode of organizing the world is today being challenged by the very voices it had silenced. These voices, muted through subjugation, are now quietly but firmly suggesting that the western male has produced only one culture, and that there are other ways of structuring the world.

—VANDANA SHIVA, *STAYING ALIVE* (2010)

PHENOMENOLOGISTS HAVE ALWAYS been Platonists, for the core of Plato's philosophy is not the metaphysics of forms valorized by Platonism, but the constant disturbance of the natural attitude. What is familiar and taken for granted hides its contingency and historicity as well as its dependencies on invisible labor and silent voices. Criticizing the images and narratives that sustain the familiar, critical phenomenology reaches for the possibility of being otherwise.

Unlike other animals, humans are not predestined by their bodies to perform a specific repertoire of tasks to ensure survival. The plasticity of the brain, hand, and foot implies that, for humans, there are multiple routes to survival, multiple sustaining forms of life. This human exceptionalism imposes on humans a particular responsibility as custodians of the generativity of the earth. How might humans collaborate with the elemental, with other animals and with plants and with each other,[1] to promote life, including human health and happiness?

Policy frequently relies on macroeconomic indicators and population variables without capturing its specific effects on the lives it affects. Perhaps a policy informed by phenomenology, a phenomenology of eating or work, for example, might be less likely to forget that, even when it is aimed at a population, policies apply themselves in the lives of individual humans and other animals as well as in the elemental itself. Policies affect lives and the conditions of living in ways that frequently escape macroeconomic or population indicators.

Putting aside the likelihood that what happens in food policy or labor policy depends more on the interests of capital and less on the nice distinctions of philosophy, debates about food policy or policies on poverty often hinge on ideas about liberty and state power. Do laws regulating sugar or fat violate liberty by restricting citizens' freedom of choice? Such debate takes for granted the current conditions and infrastructures as if they were necessary. Moreover, it deploys an entirely abstract concept of liberty, so thin as to come down to nothing more than a choice between given alternatives. Ismene demonstrates that liberty requires the physical, affective, and conceptual mobility that makes it possible to eschew a spirit of revenge in favor of a way forward. Being "at liberty" means being able to say, think, and do without fear of violence. Those who enjoy liberty are neither sold nor bartered nor raped. A citizen at liberty in the just state fears neither want nor sickness nor violence. Just food policies, universal health care, a sound pension system, and demilitarized communities and budgets would begin to realize this libertarian state.

Foucault cautions against the risk that the attempt to think otherwise will turn into a "program," conscripted by "the great political institutions and great political parties" to serve the forces of capital and biopower in maximizing wealth and security.[2] More likely, it will simply not be heard in the cacophonous space of contemporary media. Still, perhaps the invitation to *bio*ethics, to make the ethics of eating and the ethics of labor practices more central, may be heard.

Under a different captain, the crew of the *Pequod* might have enjoyed the work and learned to love and respect the prey, as many hunters do. What would happen if Ahab were no longer there to give the command? What style of leadership might be conducive to generativity and to humans' exceptional responsibility to Earth, to other living beings, and to one another? What kind of sovereignty might install and sustain collaboration among the citizens at liberty in a just state?

The whale surfaces . . .

5

Eating at the Heart
of Ethics

With the destruction of forests, water and land, we are losing our life-support systems. This destruction is taking place in the name of "development" and progress, but there must be something seriously wrong with a concept of progress that threatens survival itself. The violence to nature, which seems intrinsic to the dominant development model, is also associated with violence to women who depend on nature for drawing sustenance for themselves, their families, their societies. This violence against nature and women is built into the very mode of perceiving both. . . . Seen from the experiences of Third World women, the modes of thinking and action that pass for science and development, respectively, are not universal and humanly inclusive, as they are made out to be; modern science and development are projects of male, western origin, both historically and ideologically. They are the latest and most brutal expression of a patriarchal ideology which is threatening to annihilate nature and the entire human species.

—VANDANA SHIVA, *STAYING ALIVE* (2010)

Human activity is putting such a strain on the natural functions of the earth that its ability to maintain human well-being is now in question.

—UNITED NATIONS MILLENNIUM ECOSYSTEM ASSESSMENT (2005)

"And Man created his plants and his animals." But this "man" historically does not exist. He is an abstraction embodied in real people, who live in more or less complex societies, inside of which power struggles and conflicts for control of resources are an ongoing reality.

—MASSIMO MONTANARI, *FOOD IS CULTURE* (2004)

My people are tired of development, they just want to live.

—GUSTAVO ESTEVA, ADDRESS TO THE CONFERENCE OF THE SOCIETY FOR
INTERNATIONAL DEVELOPMENT, ROME (1985)

IN THE MYTHOLOGIES of ancient Greece, violations of the rules governing food, particularly the strictures on who is allowed to eat what or whom, result in dreadful and gruesome punishments. Prometheus convinces Zeus to allow humans to retain a portion of the sacrificed animal for their food and to commit only part to the fire dedicated to the gods. He then tricks Zeus into choosing, from the bulls he has slaughtered, the pile of bones covered in fat rather than the succulent meat hidden under the ox's hide. In his wrath, Zeus withholds fire from humans, but Prometheus steals a burning coal and delivers it to them hidden in a fennel stalk. For these offenses, Zeus condemns Prometheus to be chained to a rock in Scythia for an "agony without term." During the day, Zeus's eagle feeds on his liver "till it be black with gnawing." His liver is regenerated every night, so that the eagle may feed again.[1] All living creatures are subject to being eaten.

Tantalus stands forever in a pool in Hades. Luscious fruits hang from a tree just over his head. When he bends to drink, the waters recede. When he reaches for the fruit, the branches draw away. Some authors say that he is condemned to be thus tormented and tantalized because he made a stew of his son Pelops and tried to feed it to the gods, but Pindar and the *Library* of Apollodorus confirm that he suffers because, after being invited to Zeus' table as an honored guest, he stole ambrosia to share with humans.[2] All living creatures are subject to hunger.

Ambrosia not only refreshes, removing any sense of fatigue or weakness, it also restores the luminosity of youth and the vigor of health *in those who are immortal*. Demeter or Thetis may have tried to immortalize a specific infant by anointing him with ambrosia, and Zeus may have meant to immortalize Tantulus by setting the gods' food before him. But the liminal figure of Persephone— always at once there in the solidarity and generativity of the two mothers wrapped in the same cloak, resting after their travels, and yet also elsewhere, in her place inside the rock of the earth on the throne of the Queen of the Dead—installs the logic of life / death, and there can be no idea of immortalizing the race of humans. Like all living creatures, humans will be born, grow, age, and die. Death is immanent in human life, even if the living themselves err in making too great a distinction between the living and the dead.[3] Humans will need something other than ambrosia to eat.

The two mothers, Demeter and Persephone, figure not only the linear temporality of life / death but also the cyclical regenerative power of the seed. Each seed bears within it the infinite abyss of an impossible origin, an infinite regress of generations, but also the next generation, a material future. Iason and Dionysus taught men how to capture and domesticate animals, but women have always been the keepers of seed.[4] For ten thousand years, women and men followed the two mothers in a sustainable agriculture built around the regenerative power of the seed and the productivity of the female body.[5] Together, the mothers educated mortals about the possibilities of Earth, facilitated partnerships with other animals, and encouraged women and men to collaborate with each other, other creatures, and the elements of earth, air, and water in the nourishing and joyful pleasures of the grain and the vine.

Today, however, that collaboration is in danger. Agribusiness and biocapital threaten the generativity of the seed on which all life depends, as well as the biodiversity of Earth and the health of mortals. Unless it undertakes a critique of agribusiness, a dangerous disrespect for what nourishes life eats at the heart of ethics.[6]

Women are disproportionately responsible for food around the world, yet they are globally underrepresented in the ownership of property or decisions about land use or in determining environmental or food policy. As the spike in obesity among women and children with the shift to global food indicates, women, like other vulnerable and underrepresented populations, are disproportionately affected by globalization, as well as by environmental degradation and climate change.[7]

Women, however, are also "key drivers of change," necessary to improving food production and consumption, as well as environmental health in any community. As the Pakistani delegate to the 2007 Regional Implementation Meeting for Asia and the Pacific of the UN Commission on Sustainable Development insists, "If you pull women out, there will be no sustainable development."[8]

Research by Nussbaum and Sen, among others, demonstrates that investments in women's health improve the health of the whole community.[9]

The knowledge of women and indigenous farmers about sustainable farming and biodiversity is discounted by agribusiness and global policy institutions as "primitive" or "non-technical."[10] An appeal to science justifies the dismissal of indigenous practices in land use, water rights, and local leadership that have sustained communities for millennia. The dislocation and homogenization of food, land, and culture under globalization threatens the integrity of local cultural practices and identities to the detriment of community health. Evidence suggests that support for indigenous farming over agribusiness is more likely to promote the health and independence of the community, while many food crises in LMICs (low- and middle-income countries) can be traced to global food policy itself.[11] Many regional and international movements and statements articulate the opposition of peoples in the Global South and other nonindustrialized regions to the intrusion of agribusiness, with its devaluation and displacement of local knowledge and practice.[12]

While no human being can escape the ethical dimension of food, what and how we eat is not simply a matter of individual choice. A focus on individual responsibility ignores the dependency of human agency on a *culture of possibilities*. The philosophical approach to eating as a matter of personal virtue and choice elides the structural and historical determinants of what and how we eat, at the same time that it deflects the political strategies and collaborations necessary to install and sustain infrastructures adequate to the just production and distribution of wholesome food. As Marion Nestle argues, "The emphasis on individual choice serves the interest of the food industry for one critical reason: if diet is a matter of individual free will, then the only appropriate remedy for poor diets is education, and nutritionists should be off teaching people to take personal responsibility for their own diet and health—not how to institute societal changes that might make it easier for everyone to do so."[13] Nestle does not deny the role of "personal responsibility" in diet, but she also demonstrates how its exercise depends on "the environment of food choice." The analysis of surrogacy required attention to the infrastructures of biopower and global capital that have turned it into an economic strategy, rather than merely a focus on the individual surrogates' "choice." Similarly, a critical phenomenology of food must look beyond a thin notion of individual liberty to the food culture or environment.

Debates about state policies requiring food labeling or the regulation of sugar, fat, or salt, particularly among scholars in the United Kingdom and Australia, often refer to John Stuart Mill's famous "bridge example."[14] It appears in the context of a discussion of "how far liberty may legitimately be invaded for the prevention of crime, or of accident." The primary example is the regulation of poisons: Mill argues that warning labels, registries, and witnesses might all be required without infringing liberty, given that "the buyer cannot wish not to know that the thing he possesses has poisonous qualities."[15] Such policies make it possible to exercise liberty in obtaining the poison for legitimate use, while making it difficult to go undetected if it is used for nefarious ends. The point of the example is how far liberty may be infringed to prevent crime. In the course of the discussion of poison, Mill introduces three sentences on accidents, two on the bridge example. If a "public officer" knows for certain that a bridge is unsafe and has no time to warm someone about to cross it, he may seize the man and turn him back without any real infringement of his liberty. Conversely, "when there is not a certainty, but only a danger of mischief, no one but the person himself can judge of the sufficiency of the motive which may prompt him to incur the risk."[16] In that case, unless the agent in question "is a child, or delirious, or in some state of excitement or absorption incompatible with the full use of his reflecting faculty," the officer may only warn him, not restrain him.

There are two problems with referring to this example in debates about food and health. First, the example is flawed by its own abstraction. No one would allow a friend or lover or mother or anyone else to cross a bridge believed to present the "danger of mischief." Even if the loved one presented some urgent necessity for crossing the bridge, debate would focus on alternate strategies and avoiding the danger. Perhaps, in the end, everyone would agree that the bridge must be crossed, but not out of respect for the individual's "liberty,"[17] rather in virtue a collective decision that there was no other way. Second, the example is flawed as a reference in debates about food and eating because it is disanalogous to the situation of the individual eater in the globalized world. The man about to cross the bridge is not making a choice that is subject to global forces creating standardized options and deploying billions of dollars of sophisticated media to shape his "choice."

The dichotomy between individual choice and state paternalism on which food policy debates often turn proves doubly misleading. On the one hand, a focus on individual responsibility operates under a fiction of liberty. In LMICs, food alternatives are often severely constricted by poverty and lack of infrastructure, while in HICs (high-income countries) vast machineries of production manipulate land and water, harvest animals, and impose poor food options directly related to an epidemic of obesity and obesity-related diseases. Currently, agribusiness is expanding aggressively in LMICs with the result that, as infectious diseases decline, obesity-related diseases are spiking.

On the other hand, not only are isolated state bans on certain products unlikely to remake the culture of possibilities that determines how people eat, these bans do not represent a new intrusion of the state into the domain of food. States like the U.S. already collude with agribusiness through decades of policies favoring industrial agriculture and the economics of big farming over local sustainable farming.[18] Many states have long been complicit with agribusiness in shaping culinary practices and norms to favor global food.

The ethics of food demonstrates that, as Leibniz remarked, "everything is connected with everything else."[19] What and how we eat determines our relation to other animals, the forms of social life, the gender division of labor, and the integrity of the environment, as well as degrees of economic independence and cultural integrity under the homogenization of global capital. An ethical analysis of the basic needs binding us to each other, to other living beings, and to Earth provides the starting point for an account of justice that directly addresses gender and other systems of subjection. How would justice and ethical agency be reconfigured if eating, not property and propriety, were positioned at the heart of ethics?

EVERYTHING IS CONNECTED WITH EVERYTHING ELSE: AGRIBUSINESS, BIOCAPITAL, AND THE RIGHT TO LIFE

Farming is not adapted to large-scale operations because of the following reasons: Farming is concerned with plants and animals that live, grow, and die.
—JOEL SALATIN, POLYFACE FARMS, QUOTED IN
MICHAEL POLLAN, *THE OMNIVORE'S DILEMMA*

Proponents of global capitalism argue that agribusiness is necessary to sustain the human population in a global context. Perhaps, however, it is agribusiness itself that is unsustainable.[20] The defense of agribusiness is based on the mistaken identification of the growth of commodity production with the actual generation of health and happiness globally. In actual fact, there is less water, less fertile soil, and less genetic wealth as a result of the development process, while it displaces rural farmers and increases urban poverty. The "Green Revolution" has been linked to economic ruin for small farmers as well as spiking suicide rates in India, Sri Lanka, and China.[21]

Agribusiness threatens the seed that sustains life not only by replacing biodiversity with monoculture but also by subjecting the seed to the law of property and global capital. Seeds have traditionally circulated freely, saved by farmers, traded, and passed on. The sustainability of life depends on the generosity of the seed in yielding itself to the new plant and on the new plant generously yielding itself to be eaten, as well as to the new seed for the next plant. For millennia, this cycle of generativity sustained mortals and the animals who live with them. Now global corporations patent seeds that vary little from traditional varieties, so that peasants and indigenous farmers who continue their traditional practices become liable for fines and royalties.[22]

Even more threatening are the genetically engineered seeds that do not reproduce. These pseudoseeds will not produce fertile seed, assaulting the generativity on which life depends. They do not belong to the cycle of generation and regeneration but to the laws and interests of capital. The purpose of these seeds is to force farmers to buy annually rather than relying on gathering and trading. The strategy not only assails the cycle of regeneration on which all life depends; it transforms independent farmers into dependent consumers. It disrespects the miracle of the seed and the women's labor that has conserved it over the centuries.

The assault on the seed reflects the problem of scale cited by the grass farmer Joel Salatin. Agribusiness deploys a massive uniformity or homogenity on the land itself, as small- to mid-sized farms practicing sustainable polyculture are replaced by vast swaths of a single crop, monocultures of soy or corn that no longer support the biodiversity of the landscape. In South America and Southeast Asia, agribusiness is the primary cause of habitat destruction.[23]

The effects of scale appear in the distribution systems where small- and medium-sized businesses are swallowed by super- or megastores. In these global spaces the intimacy between producers, vendors, and consumers is destroyed, so that the history of the food eaten becomes opaque. As more and more places are overwhelmed and homogenized by the juggernaut of agribusiness, it becomes more and more difficult to take responsibility for the food that is eaten or to accord it and the labor that produces it proper respect.

The problem of scale also determines policy. Global institutions and states overwhelmingly favor agribusiness, large-scale top-down projects, and global food over smaller or indigenous farmers. The continued credibility of agribusiness, its ability to turn a profit, depends significantly on favorable government policies, particularly in the United States.[24]

Finally, the problem of scale appears on the plate, where globalization is linked to outsized portions, excess sugar and fat, and ultimately to obesity. The U.S. Centers for Disease Control estimates that 42 percent of American adults and 25 percent of American children are obese. Spiking levels of obesity in LMICs recently opened to agribusiness demonstrate the disproportions between global food and human health.

The scale of agribusiness and its disrespect for the seed threaten life by

- putting Earth itself in danger;
- disrespecting the knowledge of women and other small, nonindustrial farmers and by devaluing the labor that produces food;
- destroying the specificity of place on which the diversity of life depends;
- and by producing *malbouffe*, food that is neither wholesome and healthy nor full of flavor and pleasure.

Agribusiness poses an unsustainable threat to the generativity of Earth.

Agribusiness threatens the generativity of Earth both through the dramatic reduction of biodiversity and in its degradation of the environment or the elemental conditions of life. The scale of the assault on biodiversity is staggering: at the beginning of the twenty-first century, only 10 percent of the crops that have been cultivated in the past are still farmed.[25] A similar reduction in diversity has taken place among domesticated animals. Given its link to habitat destruction, particularly in the Global South and Southeast Asia, agribusiness is a primary force for the loss of species.

Agribusiness regularly produces unsustainable waste and environmental degradation that is inimical to life. CAFOs, or Concentrated Animal Feeding Operations, for example, impose multiple hazards that make it nearly impossible to work or live near the plants without suffering health problems and a diminished quality of life. The degradation of water and air quality in communities where CAFOs are located is associated with serious acute and chronic health problems, including headaches, respiratory ailments, diarrhea, eye irritations, fatigue, and depression. The CAFOs also subject communities to catastrophic environmental risks. "In the summer of 1995, for example, an eight-acre swine-waste lagoon in Onslow County, eastern North Carolina, collapsed, releasing approximately 25 million gallons of feces and urine into the New River. The spill polluted as much as twenty-two miles of river, causing fish kills, algal blooms, and fecal bacteria contamination."[26] This is an example of the "progress" and "development" that is killing Earth and the creatures who live on it. As Irigaray argues, we need "to grasp the idea that our species might disappear" and to begin thinking from it.[27]

With the industrialization of agriculture, the production of food shifts from a reliance on renewable and sustainable resources to inputs that must be purchased annually. Agribusiness relies on chemical rather than ecological strategies to sustain monocrop production of a handful of export-oriented and heavily subsidized commodities such as corn, soy, rice, and wheat. The hegemony of agribusiness substitutes for the genetic diversity of the planet a few monocrops that, as Michael Pollan suggests, are floating on a sea of oil.[28] By depending on monocultures, the food system, Pollan argues, is being made increasingly dependent on fossil fuels—for synthetic fertilizers, for running giant machinery, and for long-distance transportation. Pollan estimates that one acre of industrial corn requires fifty-five gallons of oil for its production: "Instead of eating exclusively from the sun, humanity now began to sip petroleum." The generic, placeless food of agribusiness consumes almost as much oil as the automobile.[29]

This reliance on fossil fuels, as well as the pollution associated with chemical inputs, makes agribusiness a chief contributor to climate change and climate degradation.[30] The evidence suggests that if humans who rely on agribusiness and global food do not change the way they eat and the way their food is produced and distributed, all living beings will be facing catastrophic changes in habitat that include drastically reduced capacities for growing healthy food.[31] The diversity of life makes a claim on us, not only because biodiversity is essential to species health but also because there is no reason to ascribe to humans any greater right to life than other species. Every form of life has the right to defend itself. What distinguishes the human is not privilege but responsibility or the capacity for respect. Transforming nature through the built environment and other forms of incursion, humans become responsible for the biodiversity that they put at risk.

Agribusiness devalues the knowledge of indigenous agricultures, as well as the labor that is required to produce food.

The scale of agribusiness makes it difficult to trace the relationship between the food eaten and the conditions of its production, while agribusiness also employs aggressive strategies to hide its practices. Strenuous efforts are made to keep the abuse of the land and animals from public consciousness.[32] This scale also alienates the one who eats from those who produce food, as if the food fell like manna from heaven. Food fails to command respect for the labor embodied in it.

The development plans of global corporations like Monsanto or ADM inevitably involve the substitution of industrialized farming methods for indigenous ones. The latter are dismissed as untested and unscientific, as if their sustainability were not a mark of the knowledge embedded in them. Global policies may or may not pay lip service to the knowledge and interests of women and other small farmers, but it is rarely the case that these farmers have a seat at the table where the decisions about global food policy are made.[33]

Agribusiness and global food retailers typically rely on nonunion contract workers.[34] The fast food produced by agribusiness is cheap, in part, because those who produce and distribute it are regularly underpaid and exploited. At the same time, this globalization of food regularly correlates with a loss of agricultural land to nonagricultural, commercial use and with increased economic dependence and dislocation for the local population. The concomitant emergence of service economies threatens the integrity of local environments, cultural practices, and landscapes, while rarely increasing the fair distribution of power and wealth. Food justice focuses on the need to reverse the disappearance of small farmers and to remedy the condition of exploited contract farmers and farmworkers, as well as the need to craft a different way to relate to the land and grow food. Ethically sustainable food requires justice in the fields and workplaces where food is produced, as well as recognition of the dignity of work and the claim to respect that is laid on us by those who grow, harvest, and prepare the food we eat.

Agribusiness, however, makes the replacement of this labor with "mechanized process" an explicit policy. Development strategies proposed by international agencies and the handful of global corporations that control agribusiness regularly note the untapped profit potential in "processing."[35] Indigenous food systems, by which unprocessed food is delivered directly from producer to consumer, are described as "primitive" and "undeveloped." By diverting that produce in order to "process" and "brand" it, the corporation extends the reach of its generic food. It disregards and destroys the durable relations between farmers, cooks, and diners, so that food no longer commands respect for the labor that produced it.

The disappearance of small farmers that results from the spread of agribusiness differentially affects women, who are overwhelmingly responsible for food production and preparation around the globe. While women in the Global South grow 60 to 80 percent of the food, they own less than 2 percent of the land.[36] Moreover, agribusiness involves a shift from women as the primary source of knowledge and skills about farming—from seed saving to composting, cultivating polycultures in the right balance, harvesting, storing, and processing—to what Vandana Shiva has called "an agriculture without women."[37] Disrespect for the labor that produces food is directly related to the dispossession of women, to their lack of economic and social agency, and to their exclusion from decisions that directly determine the future. Food sovereignty movements such as Via Campesina emphasize the rights of women farmers and embrace radical social change in the power relations between the sexes, as well as the political status of women, as a key element of agricultural policy.

In industrialized countries, "cooking tends to change genders, becoming no longer a female domestic activity but a profession exercised principally by men."[38] While the reliance on processed foods, fast foods, and restaurants has been correlated with spiking levels of obesity, particularly in the United States and other Anglophone countries, less attention has been given to the effects on happiness and sociality by the loss of the life of the kitchen and the hearth. Anthropology and history identify cooking as the "human activity par excellence."[39] The displacement of the kitchen by the fast food chain and processed food not only devalues women's traditional knowledge and labor; it also threatens identities and relationships.

Agribusiness destroys the specificity of place.

Agribusiness effects a disconnection of food from local resources that threatens the diversity of cultures around the globe. The French farmer and activist José Bové, the leader of Confédération Paysanne, coined the term *malbouffe* to describe the way global food is stripped of "taste, health, and cultural or geographical identity."[40] Agribusiness produces "food from nowhere," and the standardization of food threatens to reproduce the "same taste from one end of the world to the other."

Commodity corn serves as the generic of agribusiness and the global food industry. Not only does high fructose corn syrup regularly appear early in the list of ingredients for processed foods, but also the corn itself is cultivated in immense homogeneous tracts that sustain no other life. Diverse bioregions in the developing world are being similarly reduced to the homogeneity of soy or palm oil.

Global food reflects no place and no particular culture or history. It strives for a standardized supply and distribution chain that minimizes cultural variants. It effaces cultural difference and the specificity of tastes, even as it homogenizes the landscape.[41]

Agribusiness produces food that is unhealthy.

Malbouffe is not only placeless and a force for the erasure of place, it undermines human health. Agribusiness produces generic calories rather than genuine nutrition from diverse food sources tied to the specificity of their origin. It is directly linked to spiking levels of obesity and related diseases. Global obesity rates have doubled in the last four decades, with significantly higher rates among women and rapidly increasing rates in LMICs.[42] The "developed" world is confronted with an epidemic of obesity and related diseases, including heart disease, stroke, and diabetes. Twenty-five percent of children in the United States are obese. While the problem of obesity in HICs is well recognized, the World Bank and World Health Organization (WHO) report that, with the influx of global brands, countries like Indonesia, which still bear a heavy infectious disease burden, find noncommunicable diseases associated with obesity and poor nutrition increasing at an "alarming rate." The WHO estimates that, by the year 2020, 70 percent of diet-related disease will occur in LMICs.[43] Like many "low-income" or "developing" countries, Indonesia is in a period of "epidemiological transition." While the disease burden from communicable disease is still significant, it is in decline. At the same time, rates of noncommunicable diseases related to obesity and global food brands are spiking, especially among women and children. In a painful irony, scientists at the Indonesian Danone Institute Foundation report that undernourished children are more likely than well-nourished children to be obese as adults, linking obesity to both poverty and overconsumption.[44]

Shifts from local to global food have increased environmental hazards and subjected LMICs like Indonesia to "major issues" in food security, as well as to increases in food-related medical and dental diseases. Research by Dr. Atmarita of Gadjah Mada University in Yogyakarta indicates that, while "malnourishment exists in almost every district in Indonesia," "excessive consumption" or an "unbalanced diet" is "of growing public health importance," as "over-nutrition is a significant risk factor for a range of serious non-communicable diseases, e.g. cardiovascular disease (CVD), hypertension and stroke, diabetes mellitus, various forms of cancer, and other gastrointestinal and liver disease, and other serious health problems."[45] While the traditional Javanese diet is famously healthy, the globalization of food introduces processed foods and beverages as well as nonlocal staples that significantly undermine medical and dental health. As markets for fast food and soda flatten or decline in the rich economies, global corporations such as PepsiCo and Coca-Cola have responded by developing explicit strategies to capture markets in LMICs, undermining local food economies and agricultures as well as health.[46]

Respect for the generativity of the seed and for the labor and knowledge that have fed human beings for millennia refocuses ethics on a critique of agribusiness, paying attention to environmental integrity, to the preservation of local cultures, and to the connection between food and health as well as happiness.

Beginning with the respect due to nature's generativity and the labor, particularly women's labor, that is the condition of the food we eat, can eating and its complex infrastructures be reimagined to be more life sustaining and to better promote justice, community health, and agency for each and all? This would require that we understand how our food is produced and who has sacrificed so that we may eat.

DIFFERENTIAE: WHY EATING IS AN ETHICAL ISSUE FOR HUMANS

Tell me what you eat, and I will tell you who you are.
—JEAN ANTHELME BRILLAT-SAVARIN, *THE PHYSIOLOGY OF TASTE OR MEDITATIONS ON TRANSCENDENTAL GASTRONOMY* (1825)

Western philosophy treats the human as a perceiver and knower, not an eater and producer of waste. Food belongs to the invisible domain of women's labor and makes almost no appearance in the history of philosophy's analyses of how humans are claimed by the right or in accounts of political agency. The rhetorical strategies of rights—the fiction of the "state of nature," the myth of the voluntary social contract, the abstraction of the "person," the recreation of men in the generic Man, the ideology of equality, and the institution of fraternity as a figure of the social bond—install both a social logic that legitimates inequities of wealth and the subjection of certain classes of humans as the servants of that wealth. In particular, this economic logic not only relies on the historical status of women's bodies as the paradigm of property, whose exchange cements the bonds of fraternity, but it also requires the gender division of labor, on which, as both Hegel and Rousseau insist, the integrity of the modern nation-state depends.

This tradition of ethics and politics would have us believe that questions of ethics and political responsibility arise only after the institution of a contract that defines debts and entitlements.[47] In the state of nature, there can be no right or wrong. The rhetorical strategy of founding ethics and politics on the mythology of the state of nature and the fiction of the war of all establishes the need for the law of property, the gender division of labor, and the norms of sexual propriety. This hypothetical, mythological origin of ethics strategically denies and obscures the real phenomenological foundations of ethical relationships.

On the one hand, everyone is born of a woman and is dependent on the generativity of others. On the other hand, all mortals must eat in order to sustain life. The ethical subject is always already situated in a web of relations that embody and deploy this generativity and this nourishment. Reflection finds itself already claimed by these relations. Every mortal is indebted to the others that supply the conditions of life. Ethics begins neither with a hypothetical contract, nor with an abstract law of reason, nor with principles for maximizing happiness, but here: with the sacrifice of the other for my survival. Humans are always already indebted to the one who has nourished them and what they have eaten. No contract, law, or principle can preempt this debt that belongs to human life itself.

While plants possess the capacity to acquire their nutrients directly from the soil, sun, and water, animals must consume other living beings, either plants or other animals, to survive. For most animals, however, eating is a destiny, not an ethical challenge. As Hegel argues, the *differentiae* of a species, its tooth and claw, determine what it will eat or how it will be eaten. The beak and talon of the hawk prescribe its identity: it makes no sense to hold it accountable for eating the rabbit.

Conversely, eating poses ethical issues for human animals, because the human body does not preordain a specific mode of life. The plasticity of the human brain, hand, and foot puts identity itself in question and makes the individual responsible in who she becomes—and in what and how she eats. For the omnivorous human animal, dietary practices have ethical value because we must own them as our own.

For centuries, human beings took responsibility for what they ate, raising or killing their own food. Only very recently has it been possible for large human populations to eat without taking any responsibility for the production of their food or even without knowing where their food comes from or how it is produced. As Michael Pollan has argued, if the conditions of contemporary agribusiness were well known, it is unlikely that humans would eat as they do. Indeed, considerable resources are deployed by agribusiness and the industrial food complex to hide the circumstances under which global food is produced.

The package of chicken meat or beef in the local Western supermarket hides the traces of the procedures and techniques to which the animals have been subjected.

The aggressive efforts of Western philosophy to detach reason from the body and to misrepresent the human animal as a purely spiritual and autonomous being serve not only the installation of Man as the figure of the human but also the elision of human indebtedness to nature and to other creatures. Kant's sublime project—the mastery of nature and the mastery of nature in Man—identifies ethics with rational choice rather than with the recognition of human interdependency. This disrespect for and devaluation of what sustains human life continues to eat at the heart of ethics.

The American beef industry, for example, has effected a denaturing of the cow. Cows are destined by their very physiology to graze: they are pastoral animals, ruminants whose stomachs are constructed for the conversion of grass into flesh. Very few beef cattle in America, however, are allowed to live the life for which they are formed. Early on in their careers, these animals are transferred to CAFOs where they are fattened on corn. The physiology of cattle cannot long sustain this diet, but this strategy produces a cow ready for slaughter more quickly and efficiently than does grazing. As Michael Pollan argues, "So this is what commodity corn can do to a cow: industrialize the miracle of nature that is a ruminant, taking this sunlight-and prairie-grass-powered organism and turning it into the last thing we need: another fossil fuel machine. This one however is able to suffer."[48] Instead of lazy cows grazing in a pasture, the American beef industry produces herds that spend most of their short life hock deep in muck, eating a food entirely inappropriate to their bodies. Put aside for a moment the serious environmental pollution for which CAFOs are responsible—as Pollan notes, "They turn a precious source of fertility, cow manure, into toxic waste"— this culinary strategy denies to the animal its right to be itself, to live as a cow for as long as it lives. The cow makes a claim on us as life and through our interdependence. The cow suffers and, as Hobbes argues, is capable of the same "deliberation" as humans in avoiding harm and attaining pleasure. By domesticating the cow, humans have become responsible for it and for how it lives.

Eating responsibly requires that we know something about where our food comes from and how it is produced. It requires respect for the nature that sustains us and for the labor on which food depends. It requires that we recognize that the animals we eat are capable of suffering, and, at the very least, it requires that these animals be raised in a way that is consonant with their nature, that the cow or the chicken we eat have the opportunity to enjoy those activities and satisfactions that are particular to that animal. It is not clear to me that a global shift to vegetarianism is sustainable; moreover, such a shift would erase whole cultures and forms of life. What is clear is that eating denatured cows and chickens is ethically unsustainable. The hawk may not be responsible for the suffering of the rabbit, but we humans are thoroughly responsible for the suffering of what we eat.[49]

Scale matters. No doubt, the chickens strutting and scraping around the yard on my grandmother's farm had some vague sense that she might one day come among them, ruthless and lethal, to pluck one of their number for the Sunday dinner pot, but, for the most part, they had free run and all they needed to be chickens. They had a wooden house with small compartments, each containing a well of hay for a nest. It was my responsibility as a small girl to collect the eggs. The hens came in and out of the house at will, and, besides being constantly harassed by the two large and flamboyant roosters who pranced and swaggered around them, they pecked happily about with their delicate sense of touch for seeds, insects, and grain, as well as the small stones that would grind it all up. They loved to dust-bathe and spent hours preening. The small incubator cut into the earth about three feet deep smelled sharp and acrid with the guano of young chicks whose cheeping filled the dim and dusty air. In the spring, week by week, generations of young hens would emerge to take their place in the yard.

Perhaps my grandmother had no right to kill the hens, but we depended on them for food, and she needed to make way for the productive rearing hens that would produce the eggs she depended on for income. I have seen her do it more than once: she wrings the neck with her strong hands, then places the limp bird on a stump and cuts off its head with a small ax. She plucks it but does not dispose of the feet— they will go into the stock, along with the wing tips and fatty bits around the neck and tail.

Fresh milk, buttermilk, cream, and butter from her cows, along with the eggs, fed not only her family but also its bank account. The food we ate was not only healthy and secure, because we could trace absolutely every step of its production; it embodied an interdependence of landscape, woman, plant, and animal in which each respected and appreciated the other, even though this involved sacrifice. One day my pet pig Spare Ribs was no more, and, after a few tears, I ate the chops and ribs along with the rest of my family. We also depended on the venison from the deer my brother and father killed as well as the doves and quail they shot. They shot a wild turkey every year for Thanksgiving and for Christmas. They loved and nurtured the land and the animals that lived on it, and the land sustained them.

Every local community in this poor rural landscape had its own cookbook preserving the recipes of famous local favorites: Miss Gwen's Pound Cake, Mr. Henry's Camp Stew, or Miss Isabel's Cheese Straws. There were cookbooks from the ladies of the various churches and handbooks on barbecuing by the men's club.[50] As Montanari argues, "Invention is not born only from luxury and power but also from necessity and from poverty." The "fascination of culinary history" is to trace how humans, "with effort and imagination," have "transform[ed] the pangs of hunger and the anguish of nutritional privation into potential occasions for pleasure."[51] With neither media nor money, the women of this community turned its local bounty into satisfying and nourishing daily meals and occasional magnificent feasts.

The passage of the year seemed more marked by meals than anything else. Summer meant an abundance of tomatoes, okra, and corn. Thanksgiving brought wild turkey, cornbread stuffing, and sweet potatoes. Christmas began with quail and grits. My great aunts always served venison, but my mother, who considered it too gamey, preferred a roast from one of Mr. Henry's steers. Black-eyed peas on New Year's Day ensured good luck. Lenten Sundays were particularly festive, especially for the children, who usually had foresworn sweets for Lent and leapt at the opportunity to compensate on Sunday with the luscious array of pies and cakes that seemed to be on hand at any family gathering. The Easter Egg Hunt was always followed by my great aunt's leg of lamb and her celebrated mint jelly. As in most religious calendars across cultures, life was a series of feasts amidst a familiar routine of home cooking.

Canning and preserving were important activities requiring considerable knowledge and skill. Girolamo Sineri links canning with "anxiety in its absolute state."[52] Certainly, it is a defense against perishability, transforming abundance in the time of plenty into winter's well-stocked shelves. For several days in late summer, my mother's kitchen would be off-limits to anyone but her and her sister, a laboratory of mason jars and pressure cookers. Bushel baskets of tomatoes, beans, peas, and okra would appear regularly from the garden, courtesy of my father, and be absorbed into this alchemical enterprise. At the same time, my grandmother harvested her fig tree, planted in 1818 when her great-grandfather built the house. Hers were the only fig preserves that had the right texture and degree of sweetness. Uncharitable competitors put it down to the tree, as my grandmother, a tomboy of the outdoors, was otherwise an indifferent cook, except for an unparalleled apple pie.

My great aunts made such good pickled onions and peppers that no one else bothered. Their jellies and jams were prized goods in the family and at local fairs. The only anxiety I ever witnessed concerned the women's ability to keep up with the overwhelming abundance of the late summer harvest: they were always anxious to avoid waste. Sineri is surely right, however, when he describes canning as a "bet on the future: 'Who would ever make marmalades if he [*sic*] didn't have the hope of living at least long enough to be able to eat them?'"[53] Like all rural agricultural peoples, my family was always thinking about what needed to be done to sustain the cycles of generativity that sustained us, laboring today for the joys and pleasures of tomorrow. The women all lived well into their eighties and nineties, as did most of the men. Perhaps their longevity was genetically determined or just luck, but the locally sourced home cooking that they lived on certainly contributed to their vitality, and they surely subscribed to the ancient idea that pleasurable food is healthy food. When you were hungry for something, it was because your body needed it, and when you enjoyed something, it was because it was doing you good.[54]

Taste in this community was hardly a "subjective" matter. Not only was there general communal agreement over what tasted best, the community also shared a complex set of skills and knowledge that had been developed and transmitted over generations. As Montanari argues, "Taste is not in fact subjective and incommunicable, but rather collective and eminently communicative."[55] Considerable debate was given to every aspect of food, from which variety of corn or tomato was best to whether or not fried chicken should be battered or dusted. Tradition was required, but innovation was celebrated. When my great aunt spiked up the family barbecue sauce recipe with a new Louisiana hot sauce and replaced the brown sugar with orange juice, everyone was won over, as they were when my mother followed suit, replacing some of the sugar in the Thanksgiving sweet potatoes with orange juice and serving them in the orange shells decorated with meringue. Home cooks are infinitely inventive even as they are the keepers and transmitters of tradition.

Food was something in which to take pride and a way of showing love and honoring relationships. It cannot then go unremarked that, in a landscape where much of the labor was performed by African Americans, they did not have a seat at the table. We ate the same foods, often cooked in the same pot, but never together. We whites ate foods that African Americans had taught us to love and thought of those foods as our own. We learned from African Americans and depended on them and we organized the built environment and codes of behavior to deny them a place at the table and a part in the conversation. Only extraordinary physical courage and brilliant leadership initiated the change that is still so incomplete today. I have sometimes dared to hope that my memories of the women, black and white, standing together at the kitchen sink or counter, cooking, canning, and chatting back and forth together, might not be false. Perhaps there were moments of collaboration and respect around food on which to build.[56] Certainly, the history of Southern food in the twentieth century displays all the contradictions and injustices of two rural peoples living on the same land and eating the same food within an unsustainable legacy of slavery.

Deciding to eat responsibly cannot be reduced to a matter of individual choice. These decisions are situated in a culture of possibilities that may facilitate healthy, pleasurable, sustainable eating or may distribute *malbouffe* on a massive scale. Food may embody pleasure and community or a history of subjection. Policy often treats eating as a calculative matter of calories and nutrients, but eating always embodies a way of life, social relations, and a position in a community. These social dimensions of eating require policies that are focused on more than the point of ingestion, that take into account the complex of activities and relationships required to produce healthy and pleasurable food in a just landscape, activites and relationships that are, in turn, sustained by that food.

Agribusiness aggressively aims to regulate and constrain choice. The construction of retail space, packaging, branding, and marketing manipulate behav-

ior to produce profitable outcomes.[57] The corporations of agribusiness specifically target schools and young children in order to create brand loyalty early on.
Given the success of these practices on a global scale and the addictive quality
of foods high in sugar, salt, and fat, individual choice proves too thin to support
personal responsibility. Given the scale of the system, it is unlikely that isolated
policies limiting portions or sugar will have much effect in changing the culture
of possibilities in which human agency is actually deployed.

What can be accomplished by collective action outweighs what an individual
alone can do. What figures of ethical agency might install and sustain solidarity
in food justice and food sovereignty?

TERROIR: FOOD JUSTICE OR POLITICS OF THE SEED

The disappearance of local seeds has gone hand in hand with the disappearance
of small farmers and local food cultures. And with them, local knowledge . . .
Diversity, freedom and ensuring the potential of future evolution of agriculture
and humanity are core principles of the law of the seed.
—INTERNATIONAL COMMISSION ON THE FUTURE OF FOOD,
"MANIFESTO ON THE FUTURE OF THE SEED" (2007)

A politics of the seed begins with respect for the generativity of nature, both in
the seed and in the female body. The first guide to policy must be the promotion
and protection of this generativity as well as the nourishment of its independence or sovereignty. Neither the generativity of the seed nor of the female body
should be made subject to the laws of property and capital.

A politics of the seed respects the knowledge and labor that has sustained humans and the animals who live with them for millennia. It opposes the devaluation of that knowledge and labor in favor of global corporate or institutional
interests and the accumulation of capital. Even though women's labor has sustained agriculture, cooking, and eating for millennia, that labor has often been
and often remains invisible. As Montanari argues, "The table is a metaphor for
life, it represents . . . both membership in a group and the relationships defined

within that group."[58] Montanari conjures as his example "the differing roles among men and women in certain rural societies: the men seated at the table, the women hovering around, ready to serve, standing while eating their own meal." In fact, this effect of the gender division of labor appears across cultures where and when families still eat at home. Under a politics of the seed, women have a seat at the table. Respect for women's labor makes their exclusion from the conviviality of the feast unsustainable.

A politics of the seed recognizes the infrastructures of food as a fundamental architecture of human life. It is dedicated to changing the language and practices associated with food so that all may enjoy not only healthy but also pleasurable and interesting food, food that makes us love it and that commands our attention and respect. The knowledge of taste and the skills and techniques of cooking transform the need to eat into the enjoyment of diverse and highly articulated pleasures. Recipes, the location of the best mushrooms, batches of yeast, cups of sugar: food has always been a domain of sharing and communal pleasure. Another cook repeats a recipe, much as a scientist repeats an experiment, and with the same idea of one day going beyond it on her own to something new. She reconfirms the labor of the other cook and opens up a future of invention.

A politics of the seed is committed to the specificity of place and the diversity of habitats and to the reflection of those differences in food. It opposes the homogenization of culture and food imposed by agribusiness, even as it celebrates the "cross-pollination" and "contamination" across traditions and regions that characterizes the history of food.[59]

A politics of the seed is claimed by taste, both by the taste of flavors and by the knowledge of taste.[60] Proust links taste with memory and forgetting. While we are ordinarily caught up in our plans, taken up by the business of yesterday and tomorrow, taste focuses attention on the vivacity of immediacy. It offers a domain of sensuous discrimination equal in its forms to any other. The specificity of taste makes it, like scent, a privileged conduit for involuntary memory, an unconventionalized return of the impression of a past world. A taste that is identical to a previous taste can bring to life the entire field of sensuous experience with which its earlier impression was associated, as the taste of the madeleine dipped in chamomile tea brings back to the narrator everything that he experienced along with it in the childhood garden at Combray.[61]

Beyond these fleeting and cataclysmic moments of involuntary memory, which depend upon the rarity of a chance encounter, cheese and wine reliably offer "Le gout de la belle saison qui peut se garder jusqu'en hiver."[62] The food or wine transports us to its own time and place: a hot summer, a rainy *vendange*, a particular cave or meadow. A fresh *chèvre* tastes of the pasture in which the goats grazed, just as good Burgundy tastes of the soil in which it was grown.

Terroir refers to the way in which food and wine reflect the specificity of place in an original taste, a taste unique to that place. It encompasses both the quality and composition of soil, as well as the conditions of the specific micro-climate: the slope of the land, its drainage, and its orientation toward and exposure to the sun and wind. *Terroir* names the taste of the elemental, of Earth and the elements that sustain life. It names the taste of life.

A visitor to Burgundy cannot help but be startled by the small and fragile plots of vines that are the material origin of the great names of wine. Burgundy includes 60,000 acres of vines, compared to 235,000 in Bordeaux. The Côte d'Or includes 13,500 acres. Within that region, Bâtard-Montrachet includes 25 acres, Chevalier-Montrachet, 18.5 acres, and, the queen of these elixirs, Montrachet comprises only 19.8 acres. In autumn, at the time of the *vendange*, the vines run along the craggy hillsides in undulating rows of gold and purple, brilliant under the grey and lowering sky.

In other parts of France, such as Bordeaux, large corporate interests have taken over, so that, as is often said, at least in Burgundy, "On ne sait pas qui a fait le vin ou d'où il vient." The label on a good Burgundy will tell you where it came from and who made it. A knowledgeable reader would know from it whether the vintner was a proponent of any particular style or method and what the character of the wine was likely to be. Even large firms like Latour and Jadot make good quality wine by relying on small producers. However inscrutable the arcane rules governing the inheritance of estates in Burgundy, they have successfully prevented the displacement of local economies as well as the homogenization of the landscape, food, and social life.[63]

Similarly, the name of every French cheese "[raconte] une histoire et une géographie des paysages." Each one embodies a "dimension sociale et poétique."[64] *Terroir* names the specificity and nondisposability of place that controls not only French cuisine and eating habits, as well as French agriculture, but also the organization of space and time, the character of the built environment, the relationship between human activity and the landscape, the forms of social solidarity and collective activity, and each particular human being's own identity. A relation to food no doubt mediates every human identity, but is there any other culture where an annual competition over a ninety-cent loaf of bread could be a matter of national significance, equal to the discussion of military or economic policy in addressing the future of the nation?[65] In what other language would a consideration of the wide diversity of cheeses available be related to the question of national identity and the possibility of a unified Europe? Few countries combine successfully such thoroughgoing centralization of all human affairs with an intense and highly elaborated regionalism.[66] Food negotiates this difference: as is often remarked, the Île de France has no cheeses of its own.[67] This Leibnizian ideal of the greatest possible diversity in the greatest possible order, "cette pluralité dans l'unicité, cela plait beaucoup aux Français."[68] Yves Boutonnat, director general of the Centre interprofessionnel de documentation et d'information laitières, specifically positions cheese at the site of a national negotiation over the differences and limits of national and regional identities. Indeed, it is unlikely that any of these regional identities would have survived had not the law of the central government so carefully regulated and certified the regions' diverse and unique agricultural and vinicultural heritage.

The commitment to this food requires highly localized systems of distribution. One way of thinking about the wholesomeness of your food is to ask, "How many people have touched it?" French shopkeepers, particularly *les marchands des fruit et legumes* and *les fromagers,* become quite agitated if an unknowing customer, invariably foreign, touches the food before buying it. When I buy a zucchini in an American supermarket, it is invariably a bit worn looking, bruised and marked, because it has been so frequently handled by any customer who would. When I buy a zucchini in France, its smooth, unblemished skin supports the confidence that no one has touched it save the producers and the greengrocer himself.

The national commitment to this food depends not only on preserving the landscapes necessary to produce it but also on complex bodies of knowledge and elaborate social rituals and institutions. The greengrocer, like the *caviste* or *fromager,* prides himself on his knowledge: when I ask for a melon, he wants to know when I will eat it, and he picks the one that will be ripe at the right moment. Smelling, tapping, touching, he picks out the fruits, vegetables, and herbs with the authority of a lifetime spent getting to know them. The injunction against touching might seem precious to the unknowledgeable foreigner, but it preserves the wholesomeness and taste of the food at the same time that it shows respect for the knowledge of the greengrocer. Indeed, the choosing of fruits and vegetables becomes an intensely social act, a theater of exchange not only for knowledge but for performing character as well. The combination of imperious judgment and respect that my tall, red-haired Australian goddaughter Madeleine employs, in her perfect French, to charm my greengrocer elicits from him a nimble dance of attention, as he hurries into the back of the store for something special for Mademoiselle—a little theater that becomes a family story of joy and character.

In this environment a curious foreigner, willing if ignorant, is quickly adopted as a pupil. Trying to buy a wine on a budget of ten Euros, the customer is quizzed about what she is serving and how it is being cooked. Shrimp? Red or grey? Prepared how? No one grills me like *le boucher*, who seems slightly offended by the idea of selling me his meat, so little confidence does he have in my ability to appreciate it and treat it properly. "Madame, [Gallic sneer] il faut ne pas trop cuisiner."

The *fromager* is kinder. Having perceived early on both my ignorance and my fondness for fresh *chèvre*, he simply works his way across France and the long shelves lining his narrow shop, offering first one cheese and then another, each one a "little tour" of its eponymous region, village, or farm. Small white cylinders, sometimes sweet, sometimes pungent; flat pucks dusted in ashes, stark white, crumbly and earthy on the inside; piquant little pears pierced with tiny sticks; pyramids with chalky white interiors that taste of grass and stones. Creamy cheeses wrapped in chestnut leaves or soaked in marc or nestled in a little earthenware dish. Hard cheeses like a gritty Vieux Comté or soft melting cheeses like a Camembert *fermier.* The poetic language of French cheeses evokes not only history and place but also a whole set of decisions that determine the specific identity of each cheese. Pont-L'Eveque was already celebrated for its cheese when Guillaume de Lorris praised it in *Le Roman de la rose* (1230). Shaped like a small book, the cheese is arrayed on shelves for its *affinage* or ripening, so that the *cave d'affinage* looks like a small library. Morbier is marked by the streak of ash through its golden flesh. To test the ripeness of Langres, you must take the measure of the depth of its sunken top: "plus la cuvette est profonde, plus il est affiné." Fat round *boules* of mimolette are brushed to aid respiration and tapped to test aging. Le Puligny Saint Pierre takes its name from the tower that also gives it its form. It must be worked by hand and must drain for at least twenty-four hours. It must rest seventy-two hours after being turned out of its mold and dusted with white salt before beginning its *affinage*. The cylinder of Saint-Maure de Touraine must be pierced through the heart with a piece of straw. Chaource and Cabicou, Picadon and Saint Nectaire; Tomme de Savoie and Selle sur cher: over 450 officially recognized cheeses, about sixty under the system of controlled names, along with hundreds of other local varieties, comprise a veritable botanical kingdom of cheese, as various and ordered as any phylum in nature, with its unpredictable identities and unmistakable kinships.[69] A humanbody might nobly devote her one life to this art.

The food demands an intellectual commitment. One must know something, as all the food embodies a specific origin, a *traçabilité*. It takes a certain amount of temerity to pronounce on a wine or a cheese in a French setting. The remark will certainly elicit conversation and, most likely, debate, even among youth. The average French person has a sufficient knowledge of the variety and complexity of wine and cheese to be proud of her own experience and expertise as well as clearly aware of its limits. An intelligent assessment of the hundreds of French cheeses would require knowledge of the history and geography of each one, of the particular herd that is the origin of its milk, the methods of preparation and aging specific to it, as well as its proper appearance and taste and the particular way it should be eaten. Some cheeses are heated; some are eaten with a spoon; some thinly sliced or spread or eaten whole.

Now there is always an intellectual element to good food: my mother's pound cake embodied considerable know-how, as did my father's barbecued ribs, but the French have made food a field of analysis and a space of discourse. Each taste has been analyzed, catalogued, and set in relation to other tastes. All sorts of collective practices and institutions have grown up around these gustatory treasures, so that the experience of them comes to organize and permeate the rest of life. The Hospice de Beaune or the syndicates of the various cheeses are not only business entities but deeply resonant cultural institutions that organize a variety of regions of life, social, economic, and political. As André Malraux remarked, in France a birth, death, or marriage is just an occasion for a good meal.

Eating this food requires attention and takes time. The point of eating is not the satisfaction of an appetite so blunt as to be content with mere bulk; indeed, portions are intentionally modest, so that an unpleasant fullness will not accompany the experience of a range of tastes. The aim of eating this food is the taste, which must be savored and tarried with if it is to be understood, appreciated, and discussed. "Ironically, although the French eat less than Americans, they seem to eat for a longer period of time, and hence have more food experience. The French can have their cake and eat it as well."[70] The French enjoy greater pleasure in their food, at the same time that their culinary habits make them healthier.[71] This food makes ethical claims and teaches certain attitudes. It requires attention not only in its preparation but also in its enjoyment, which could never be reduced to something so generic as a logic of consumption. It takes attention to distinguish and relate a complicated palette of tastes and textures. It takes patience to prepare the food: neither my mother's pound cake nor a *blanquette de veau* will be hurried. It takes time also to savor this food. Some tastes and textures, sweetbreads or *pied de cochon* perhaps, may require time to educate the palate to their particular pleasures.

Preparing this food takes even more time, but it rewards the cook with the infinitely various smells, tastes, and textures of the kitchen. Grinding fragrant spices, crushing pungent cloves of garlic, chopping onions to release their eye-watering sharpness, grating, shredding, slicing, dicing: cut determines taste by texture and by releasing the flavors differently in each case. A good stew is not made by throwing everything into the pot at once. There will be a stock of bones and roots made earlier. The meat will be sautéed separately, as will most of the vegetables. Cooking will allow their flavors to interpenetrate while remaining distinct. The stew rewards the cook with the increasing intensity and richness of its broth that, strained and enriched, will become a sauce. The sweet smell of yeast rewards the baker, as does the magical transformation of the sticky mess of flour and liquid into the silky-smooth dough, ready to rise. Knead with the heel of the hand and pull back, over and over, until the dough is smooth and almost shiny. In two hours, it puffs itself up: children love to punch down the slightly crusty top and take over on the final brief kneading and shaping. The whole house smells of bread.

The specificity of food is linked not only to particular places but also to particular times. Throughout the year, merchants announce that something *est arrivé*. Every food has its epoch, every epoch its food: white asparagus in the spring; Beaujolais and truffles in the fall. Each merchant presses you to buy what is in season or at its best, as one should taste every food in its own time. The food that graces the table reflects the passage of time and the change of climates throughout the year. The cycle of feasts provides the infrastructure of time no less than do the cycles of nature.

Those who produce and sell this food expect you to give it its due: to prepare it properly, to eat it with savor, attention, and appreciation, and to waste nothing. Like most essentially rural peoples, the French eat every part of the animals they slaughter, "head to toe."[72] They have dozens of recipes for stale bread and buy their vegetables daily in the amounts needed. The chicken carcass is the base of the stock that will flavor the next stew, and the shells of the crustaceans are essential to the richness and briny undertones of any good *bisque*. This cultural allergy to waste displays respect for the food and the labor it embodies. Food claims respect because of what has been sacrificed to the satisfaction, nourishment, and joy of the diner. Humans become responsible for what they eat: obliged to treat it well and to enjoy it. The joys of cooking and taste command attention and take time, and it takes time to repay the generosity of Earth and the labor that turned the elemental into a meal.

The intricate interlacing of a landscape of domesticated animals and plants with the production of food, eating habits, agricultural and economic institutions, and forms of social life supports and requires attention, at every level and in every register, to the sacred dimension of eating, to the extraordinary gustatory range and precision of the human tongue, as well as to the infinite inventiveness of generations of cooks. It requires respect for and homage to what is being sacrificed. Overcooking the meat or drinking cola with the langoustine is offensive because it disrespects what has given itself to the needs of your body and the possibilities of your palate. What is wasted or unappreciated is not itself waste but something of intrinsic value that makes an ethical as well as an aesthetic claim on us. Disrespect for what and who nourishes human life eats at the heart of ethics.

Situating eating at the heart of ethics resituates humanbodies in a culture of relations that promotes health, pleasure, and social life as well as the health of

Earth, the elements, and the other animals with whom we share this landscape. Food makes a claim on us to respect and protect the generativity of Earth and its elements. Unlike the homogeneous processed products and generic taste of industrial agriculture, the food of *terroir*, whether in France or Alabama, commands humans to respect taste, both the sensuous precision of the human tongue and the social life, cultures, and knowledges that have grown up around it. This food lays a claim on those who eat to respect the labor that brought the food to the table.

◆ ◆ ◆ ◆

Ten thousand years ago, men and women followed Demeter and Persephone, learning to nourish themselves while respecting Earth, and the elements of air, water, and fire on which all living beings, plant and animal, depend. The two mothers wrapped in the same cloak, one representing the cyclical renewal of the seasons, the other the linear temporality of the living being who is born, ages, and dies: together they represent this double logic of life and death, life and re-generation, but they are also a figure of solidarity and collaboration. Demeter will not give up her daughter, and she defeats Zeus to get her back. Persephone will not acquiesce: even though she is willing to play her part in the drama of mortality, she will not be separated from her mother. Together, they walk far, teaching mortals how to collaborate with the earth and other animals, how to enjoy the grain and the vine. At the end of the day's labors, they sit together wrapped in the same cloak, leaning upon and toward one another, in a perfect poise of constancy and confidence.

The food produced by agribusiness is nutritionally corrupt, ethically corrupt, and environmentally corrupt. Our collective dependence on it is neither nec-essary nor sustainable. We could learn to feed ourselves differently from those "primitive" farmers and cooks who celebrate the local, sustainable, and specific. If we fail to eliminate agribusiness and do not learn to feed ourselves differently, perhaps from those "primitive" farmers and cooks, we will continue down a deadly path of pandemic disease, environmental degradation, and social injus-tice, but not for long.

6

A Working Life

The poor person does not exist as an inescapable fact of destiny. His or her existence is not politically neutral, and it is not ethically innocent. The poor are a by-product of the system in which we live and for which we are responsible. They are marginalized by our social and cultural world. They are the oppressed, exploited proletariat, robbed of the fruit of their labor and despoiled of their humanity. Hence the poverty of the poor is not a call to generous relief action, but a demand that we go and build a different social order.

—GUSTAVO GUTIÉRREZ, *THE POWER OF THE POOR IN HISTORY* (2004)

We hold these truths to be self-evident, that all men . . . are endowed . . . with certain unalienable Rights, that among these are Life, Liberty and the pursuit of Happiness—That to secure these rights, Governments are instituted among Men, deriving their just powers from the consent of the governed.

—U.S. DECLARATION OF INDEPENDENCE (1776)

SINCE HOBBES, A man's worth has been determined by his "price" on the open market: "The *Value,* or Worth of a man, is as of all other things, his Price, that is to say so much as would be given for the use of his Power."[1] Like all animals, humans must labor for their survival. Among humans, however, just as words become forces provoking appetite and fear, so too labor becomes a satisfying good traded on the market. At the very moment that Man secures the right to property and the fraternity of citizens through the installation of the social contract, he finds himself required to sell his labor. While the sovereign is obliged to secure peace and adjudicate conflict, he is not obliged to care for the citizen, who must labor to feed, clothe, and house himself and the subjects of his "little Monarchy." While examples exist of trades or businesses handed down from father to son, most humans today face the task of figuring out how to make a life work or, the same question, how to make a life's work.

Plato makes work central to the just state and the condition of personal identity.

More than two thousand years later, Franklin Roosevelt does the same, backing up the theory with policy strategies and political leadership. Instead of situating identity in the oedipal narrative of fraternal and paternal violence or the narrative of nature as war, Plato and Roosevelt make identity contingent on collaboration in a just state through meaningful work. Their politics of work, as well as the differences in their positions, directly address the contemporary global crisis of exploited labor.

In the twenty-first century, the post–World War II collaboration between labor and capital that built a thriving middle class in the United States and Europe has unraveled. Developing nations and the global corporations that locate in them depend on cheap, unregulated, unorganized labor as part of their economic strategy and business model. While macroeconomic indicators show gains in per capita income in the LMICs, social inequity is widening in these economies. At the same time, labor in Anglo-European countries, particularly in the United States, has come under severe pressure to keep wages down and cut benefits. Part-time employment increasingly replaces full-time work. New software allows companies to calibrate staff to demand in real time, so that low-wage part-time workers find themselves "on call" for long periods. These factors exacerbate the unsustainable gender division of labor.[2] Without infrastructures to support the integration of work and family or the reliability and benefits of full-time employment, the conditions of possibility for identity, for a happy and healthy life of meaningful work, do not exist. When economic recovery and growth fail to yield significant progress toward full employment, state power appears to be all on the side of capital. There seems to be no effective counter-force to the narrative that what is good for the rich is good for all or at least that it is their due—just as poverty is the due of the poor.

It was not always so.

On January 6, 1941, eleven months before the bombing of Pearl Harbor, with Hitler in possession of Europe, imperialism expanding around the globe from South Asia and China to Latin America, and the massacre of six million Jews well underway, Franklin Roosevelt delivered an unprecedented third inaugural address to a United States Congress and a country that still hoped to avoid going to war against fascism and Nazism. A people with a tradition of noninvolvement, who sent soldiers to the distant slaughter of World War I only to see the same corrupt imperialist and colonialist powers arise again afterward like a reshuffled deck, might not be inclined toward a new involvement in international affairs, in Europe or anywhere else. A people who had barely begun to emerge from what would prove to be the worst economic catastrophe of their century might be forgiven for being unready to assume the costs and rigors of war, however necessary the cause. A politician, calculating votes, might have been expected to talk of peace and the need for negotiation or to strike an isolationist tone by focusing on domestic issues, assuming a silence on international affairs that Roosevelt's contemporaries would have found neither unusual nor disturbing.

Instead, in what has come to be known as the "Four Freedoms Speech," Roosevelt announces a moment "unique" in American history, when "our actions and our policies" should be devoted "exclusively" to foreign affairs, "for all our domestic problems are now a part of the great emergency."[3] The speech foresees a globalized world, which, Roosevelt insists, is coming in some form, no matter what. Isolationism will be impossible. The survival of the American republic, Roosevelt argues, will depend on the character of the relations that bind it to foreign powers.

Roosevelt foresees, on the one hand, the "dictator's peace" in which "law lacks mutuality in its observance" and therefore becomes an "instrument of oppression" in a world without freedom of expression or religion. The aggressive tyrant who rules by fear and violence waits only for a tactical advantage to launch his attack. Roosevelt reinscribes the unsteady peace Americans hoped to sustain as unreadiness before an inevitable assault. As Hobbes argued, a state of war exists, even without actual conflict, when the disposition to fight makes war inevitable.[4] Peace is impossible with tyrants and dictators, because they will always resort to force to secure their authority and interest. Roosevelt tells his listeners not only that they must go to war, but that they are already at war in all but the formal declaration and actual attack.

On the other hand, he lays out a "vision" of genuine peace for Congress and the American people. Roosevelt reimagines basic infrastructures of life in America in order to secure the health and happiness of its citizens. In his vision, justice as well as security and freedom depend on full employment and on securing the conditions under which each citizen can flourish in meaningful work. Issuing a call to action, he articulates a list of specific policies that need to be enacted in order to free citizens from fear so that they are free for the "joy" of meaningful work.

Roosevelt locates these domestic concerns, however, in an international frame. A republic of free citizens, if it wishes to survive, must seek a world of other such free republics. The "antithesis" of the world of tyranny, where power sustains itself through fear, propaganda, and violence, a community of free nations exists on "international generosity" and constitutes "the return of true independence." The realization of this world of free nations bound by reciprocity and respect depends, Roosevelt argues, on the achievement of full employment "everywhere in the world." From his first inaugural address in 1933, Roosevelt develops an analysis of work as the locus of freedom and happiness. Collaborating toward a world where everyone has an equal opportunity to find the "joy of achievement" in meaningful work, Roosevelt insists, is not only necessary to international security and liberty, it is "even good business."[5]

GLOBAL INEQUITY: INVISIBLE LABOR, BLIND CONSUMERS, AND THE MYTH OF THE "FREE MARKET"

Michael Pollan argues that if "consumers" in the United States knew how their food was produced, they would not eat it.[6] Consumer "ignorance" features as an essential ingredient in the business model of industrial agriculture. A similar blindness proves essential to labor practices under globalization.

To some degree, the exposure of abusive labor conditions, as well as related catastrophes and loss of life, puts pressure on large global corporations to improve labor practices in developing countries like Bangladesh or China. What remains invisible to the consumer in the smartphone or clothing that he purchases is that the exploitation of cheap labor in emerging economies is essential to globalization, not an exceptional circumstance that might be remedied. Invisible in these products, as well, is the evisceration under globalization of the postwar contract between labor, business, and the state that yielded unprecedented increases in social equity and mobility in the United States and Europe.

The cheaper products touted by globalization as its chief justification regularly hide costs both to the health and security of labor and to the environment. Global agribusiness, for example, justifies itself by its cheap prices, at the same time that it aggressively hides its conditions of production. In the United States agribusiness has successfully lobbied to block investigative reporting on CAFOs and other industrialized animal farming operations, so that the public is uninformed about the maltreatment of animals as well as the serious environmental risks posed by these operations.[7] The health threat posed by the wide use of antibiotics in industrial animal operations is not visible in the consumer's burger. The threat to the environment from agribusiness' reliance on artificially cheap and highly polluting fossil fuel consumed in producing its fertilizers and in its transportation is not visible in the consumer's fast food. Consumers see only the immediate price tag, and the real costs of globalized production to labor, to the environment, and to citizens' health remain invisible. Due to this blindness, the citizen becomes complicit in the very system that exploits him as consumer and as laborer.

In both developing and developed countries, globalization has produced widening social inequity. The structural inequity associated with globalization results not from differences in individual effort or talent but from features of the economic and political systems themselves, which favor the concentration of privilege and wealth. Hobbes described money as the "ensanguination" of the body politic: it must circulate freely to all members if the body is to be healthy.[8] The contemporary global financial system thrives on a metaphorics of free circulation. Its markets, however, favor capital, not labor, so that a very small percentage of the population owns a rapidly increasing share of resources. In the United States 35.4 percent of wealth is owned by the top 1 percent. The bottom 80 percent own 11.1 percent of wealth. The wealth of the bottom 80 percent has decreased by 7.7 percent since 1983.[9] In 2006 the United Nations' World Institute for Development Economics Research reported that 10 percent of the world's population owns 85 percent of its wealth, while the poorest 50 percent own just 1 percent. "Free" markets are, in fact, highly regulated and subsidized to serve this concentration of capital and are accessible only to privilege. Ordinary citizens, who have been led to think of themselves as "investors," have neither the information nor the scale of capital to compete successfully in these markets.[10] Once vital communities find themselves the necrosing members of a body politic whose sanguination has been cut off or dammed up, whose life fluid does not flow freely throughout.

Public policy analysis that relies on macroeconomic indicators operates at a scale under which the real effects of policy on ordinary citizens remain invisible. Measures of GNP may indicate "growth," but they are sufficiently aggregated to hide concentrations of privilege and wealth or increases in social inequity. As Martha Nussbaum remarks, the GNP "fails to provide an adequate basis for normative thinking in large part because it is not individualistic enough: it does not look at people one by one to see how each one is doing."[11] Macroeconomic indicators or analyses that focus on aggregated classes or social units make invisible the real conditions of experience for specific individuals. In treating the family as a basic social unit and basing evaluations of welfare on its economy, public policy and economic analysis can remain blind both to the systematic deprivations women may endure in the family structure (less food, less education, less health care) and to the positive contributions of their labor to the welfare of the family and community.

Drawing a distinction between development and growth, Amartya Sen argues that, while an expansion of GNP, other things being equal, should enhance the living conditions of people, there are, in fact, always other variables that determine those conditions. Things are never equal. Growth under globalization is rarely distributed equally across income groups. "It is possible . . . for a country to have an expansion of GNP per head while its distribution becomes more unequal, possibly even the poorest groups going down absolutely in terms of their own real incomes." Sen notes the necessity for looking at income distributions in relation to racial, regional, and class groups, a list to which sexual difference should be added, as Sen acknowledges elsewhere.[12] The growth of the global economy both increases inequity and inflicts heavy costs on the least well off, such as displacement or forced migration and the dispossession of traditional homes, lands, and practices.[13]

Sen also demonstrates how many benefits and costs remain invisible to the market. He notes the lack of recognition of environmental costs or the underpricing of natural resources in market calculations. He might also have noted the failure to count the benefit of domestic and agricultural labor performed predominately by women. This labor remains invisible to GNP and other macroeconomic indicators. As Vandana Shiva argues, "Growth in the global economy has led to the destruction of nature's economy—through which environmental regeneration takes place. It has also destroyed the people's sustenance economy—within which women work to sustain society. Ironically, this hard, unpaid labor is frequently denied the name of work."[14] The degradation of nature's generativity and the invisibility and discounting of the generative labor of women are not separate problems, but symptoms of the same biopolitical structure of inequity. In Shiva's analysis, macroeconomic actors, such as the World Bank and WTO, regularly favor large multinational corporate interests at the expense of the local, "informal" economy, particularly small farmers who are mostly women.[15] While failing to calculate the environmental costs of agribusiness, or the cost of its extensive subsidies, or the cost of the artificially low priced nonrenewable energy on which it depends, these global agents, at the same time, measure wealth, growth, and economic productivity in ways that ignore or underestimate the benefits of women's generative labor in the home and the field or the informal economies it sustains.[16] The methodologies used by these agents of global capital to measure "growth" are complicit with the system of inequity that increasingly concentrates wealth and privilege in the hands of a few.

The "structural reforms" required of developing countries by these agents of globalization invariably land most heavily on the poor and tend to fall disproportionately on women and children, as these policies consist largely in eliminating or reducing funding for education, health care, food subsidies, unemployment benefits, and other programs aimed at addressing social inequity and promoting upward mobility.[17] In developed countries, researchers have chronicled the struggle of women to support themselves and their children in the minimum wage and part-time employment that is available to them under globalization.[18] Globally, economic distress regularly leads women to the sex trade as a means of survival. In an environment where the value of anything is determined by money, humanbodies, mostly women and girls, become commodities to be bought and sold in well-developed global markets.[19] Sex trafficking is the most common form of modern-day slavery, and its victims are overwhelmingly women and girls. No woman really wants to do this work, to turn the intimacy of her generativity into degrading violence.[20]

Under globalization, labor, particularly women's labor, is discounted and disempowered, even invisible. The eleven hundred Bangladeshis, mostly women, who died in the Rana Plaza disaster were invisible to consumers while they were inside the factory making clothing for Benetton or Primark. Their horrific working conditions and poor compensation were invisible in the clothing marketed to Western consumers until the factory building collapsed. A brief outrage follows, along with a promise by complicit companies to do better, but these commitments quickly fade, as the exploitation of this labor is essential to the economics of globalization.[21] What lies behind the label Made in Bangladesh or Made in China must remain invisible. The conditions under which workers make the T-shirts and smartphones of globalization would be intolerable to the consumers who buy these products.

The economic mobility afforded by globalization belongs to capital, not to labor. Global corporations move factories from countries where labor, through collective bargaining, enjoys rights and benefits, to countries where labor has few if any rights and little bargaining power. The global labor market is characterized by low pay, abusively long hours, a failure to pay for overtime, dangerous working conditions, surveillance, and physical intimidation or abuse. Complaints or attempts to organize are regularly punished by beatings or other physical threats.[22] When these practices come to light through investigative reporting or a catastrophe like the Rana Plaza collapse, companies address the public relations problem, but little seems to change for the garment workers themselves. The purpose of moving to Bangladesh was to cut costs, so that products can remain cheap and profit margins high. If workers in Bangladesh or China enjoyed the same safety rules and benefits as an American worker, the factories would still be in Detroit or Pittsburgh. The business model of these factories, like the business model of the private / public partnership of the Indian surrogacy clinics, depends on a steady supply of this vulnerable, disrespected, and disenfranchised labor. The economic model of globalization depends on consumers' blindness both to the exploited labor embodied in the products they buy and to the way in which their own identity as workers and the world of labor itself is threatened by globalization's reliance on renewable pools of cheap, unprotected, and unorganized labor.

Globalization exacts invisible costs on ordinary citizens that do not figure in its accounts of "growth." It is associated with environmental degradation and health risks, as well as increasing inequity, physical and social displacement, and economic dependence. While pretending to advance the free circulation of ideas, goods, persons, and wealth, globalization produces widening social inequity, forced migrations and confinements, and workers who, whether documented or undocumented, cannot expect institutions and policies that reflect respect for their labor. Globalization can supply neither the "international generosity" nor the forms of transnational collaboration that Roosevelt foresaw as necessary both to security and prosperity. As Peter Buffett insists, justice requires "concepts that shatter current structures and systems." Justice requires reconfiguring the relation of labor and the state, not by pursuing isolationism or barriers to genuinely free trade, but by exposing the deceptions of globalization's metaphorics of "growth" and "free circulation," its threats to the environment and human health, and its devaluation of labor, particularly the generative labor of women. Such a critique opens the way for a concept of justice based on respect for labor.

LABOR AND THE JUST STATE

"With one little accounting trick, I can make more money for the company than all your new furniture designs put together."
—LOREN PHINEAS SHAW (FREDRIC MARCH), *EXECUTIVE SUITE* (1954)

Both Plato and Roosevelt define justice in the state in relation to the labor of each citizen. For Plato, justice is a matter of "minding one's own business" in the sense of performing on behalf of the community the tasks, actions, or services to which the citizen's particular talents are suited.[23] Each citizen, Plato argues, will be healthier and happier engaged in pursuits that are both appropriate to his or her endowments and clearly appreciated by the community as worthwhile. The just state's twofold duty is to ensure the security of its citizens and to educate them properly so that their talents are discovered, developed, and deployed for the benefit of all.

For Plato, the most serious impediment to attaining justice in the state is *pleonexia*, a kind of greediness in which the citizen fails to stick to his own business. Such a citizen arrogates to himself an authority that properly belongs to others. *Pleonexia* may take many forms, as when an unqualified politician seeks higher office or a poor craftsman makes rickety tables. They attempt tasks for which they lack the requisite skills or abilities, with unfortunate results for all.[24]

The most serious form of *pleonexia*, however, arises from a confusion around money. Using medicine as his example, Plato argues that when a physician puts "moneymaking" above patient care, he ceases to be a physician. Injustice results when one fails to mind one's own business by substituting the aim of making money for the true aim of excelling in one's appropriate labor. Labor that alienates itself from its own task in favor of profit will prove unhappy, for itself and for its community.

On Plato's analysis, labor, unlike money, has intrinsic value and commands respect because it is productive of the good in every register of life: a clean, safe street bustling with life; a cured patient; a steady table. Meaningful work promotes the flourishing of the worker and her community by adding value. Virtually every good, except the beauty of nature and the laughter of children, is the result of some worker's industry. Labor is good for the laborer as it allows her to realize her talents and become who she is, assuming that she knows and minds her own business. Justice depends on an educational program adequate to identify and nourish the true labor of each and all. Health and happiness are generated by minding one's own business in a state where everyone else is doing so too.

Having secured its citizens' safety, the primary task of the just state is to install an educational program adequate to identify and nourish the gifts of each and all. In book 5 of the *Republic*, Plato argues that every citizen should have an equal access to the education necessary for her to flourish as a laborer in the collaborations of the community. This identification of citizenship with meaningful work trumps even the prejudices of gender. At a time when women were considered property and confined to domestic spaces and the care of the body, Plato's Socrates argues that, because some women are smarter or stronger than some men, citizens must be judged according to their talents and capacities, not their sex. Some women will make better warriors or scientists or even philosophers than some men. It is the task of the educational system to make these identifications and to nourish each citizen according to her own talents.

Plato also insists on the elimination of private property and on the dissolution of the family as the locus of private property to ensure that each member of the state identifies himself with the whole community, rather than some part or faction. In the just state, where each citizen minds her own business, you are what you do. A citizen's value is not his "Price" in a market, but his capacity to contribute to the health and happiness of the whole. Justice in the state requires recognition of and respect for the labor of each and all. To respect means to see in the mode of "looking back."[25] Justice requires that I see the worker in the dress that I wear or the meal that I eat. The other worker looks back at me in her work, and I am obliged to acknowledge that vision by looking back. The cashier or the cleaner or the cabbie is not just a functionary or a cost factor in a production line. Labor, even when it is paid, is a gift on which the community depends. Competence, reliability, enthusiasm, and loyalty are all forms of the generosity of labor. Each citizen in the just state labors for herself and for all. Each citizen enjoys, with other citizens, a reciprocal relation of "looking back" as they collaborate toward the mutual ends of health and happiness. The invisibility of labor under global capital violates this ethical requirement and facilitates its material mistreatment and disenfranchisement.

To the extent that the excellence of her labor is compromised by the aim of making money, the citizen ceases to be who she is and disturbs the whole community with degraded work. An opera singer may select one engagement over another because of a larger fee, but to the extent that the choice requires an aesthetic compromise, she demeans herself and deprives the community of her special contribution. When a legislator votes for one bill and not for another because he is serving the interest of campaign contributors, he abdicates his authority to govern in the name of the people. He substitutes the expedient for the right, and the people suffer for it through lax regulation or expensive subsidies. When a physician pays more attention to turnover rates and revenue generated than to the specificity of each patient, he elevates moneymaking over his medical labor and the good it serves. While making money may not be bad, taking moneymaking as an aim in itself tends to corrupt the real work.

Under globalization, the most spectacular wealth accrues to those who perform no labor whatsoever, except moneymaking or gambling in the markets. The hedge fund manager or investment banker works for no one except himself and his privileged clients, and he produces nothing but monetary wealth or credit with the house. Yet his wealth is vast in proportion to most workers.

Under globalization, corporations are judged not by the excellence of their product or service but by their stock price and market share. Excellence and share price may be related, but the former is regularly sacrificed to the latter. Moreover, when moneymaking is privileged as the paradigm of productive activity, labor is transformed from a positive value, commanding collective respect, as in Plato's just state, to a cost to be "kept down" and "contained" as much as possible. In the last four decades, in the developed world, particularly in Britain and the United States, a relentless assault on labor has left most workers with stagnant wages, no pensions, and rapidly eroding, if any, benefits. Only at the upper reaches of the pay scale, in the thin crust of upper management, do salaries, bonuses, and perquisites seem capable of inflating infinitely.

Plato thought that minding your own business would generate a hierarchy of expertise in which the best ruled, and each citizen labored for himself and all. The educational system, not democracy or the market, would determine one's place in the order. Plato envisions a ruling power that descends vertically, controlling freedom of both expression and religion in order to cultivate communal commitment and an identification with the state over personal interest. Nussbaum suggests that Plato's analysis, or at least Platonism, proves inadequate as a theory of justice insofar as it gives little credit to the knowledge of experience.[26] Even if Plato does recognize perception and craft as forms of knowledge, he values stability over creativity and does not see how knowledge might be generated and circulate horizontally through collaboration rather than vertically through authority. Moreover, while experience may be a source of knowledge, a strict hierarchy of experiences means that knowledge and authority are concentrated with a privileged few. All experience is valuable, but some much more than others. The knowledge of farming and cooking does not rank with the knowledge of the warrior or statesman, as if the former could not productively inform the latter.

Like Plato, Roosevelt takes the productive employment of a well-educated labor force to be the central mission of a just state, but he embraces freedom of expression and religion as essential to justice as well as to the creativity and initiative that make "good business." Instead of concentrating authority and privilege in an elect few, Roosevelt invests authority in democratic processes and in "the hands and heads and hearts of ... millions of free men and women."[27] What citizens love and what they can do is as important as what they think. In Roosevelt's vision, the knowledge of heart and hand informs thought and judgment, especially in public policy. Policy should promote a "civilized society" collaborating toward health and happiness. Like Ismene, Roosevelt eschews hardheadedness and hardheartedness for the fluidity of thought and feeling that makes collaboration possible and the future sustainable.

Of the "basic things" a citizen can justly expect of the state, the most important are "equality of opportunity" and "jobs for those who can work." Roosevelt recognizes that the prosperity and stability of the state depend on securing these aims. "The inner and abiding strength of our economic and political systems is dependent upon the degree to which they fulfill these expectations." Unemployment is a prima facie indictment of the state's injustice, as well as a threat to its security and to the health and happiness of its citizens.

Taking full employment as the standard of the just state, Roosevelt takes aim at the financial interests that would undermine it. The health of the just state is properly measured not by growth in GNP but by its ability to facilitate those collaborations that will secure the welfare of its citizens. Companies that exploit differences in wages and benefits to reduce labor costs or corporations that exploit tax law to shelter profits are not only "bad for business," to the extent that they serve the concentration of wealth and privilege rather than the free circulation of knowledge and goods, but, in Roosevelt's view, are also deeply unpatriotic. He warns against a "small group of selfish men who would clip the wings of the American eagle in order to feather their own nests." He foresees how the concentration of wealth and privilege threatens justice by devaluing the work of the many in favor of the interests of the few. If, as Peter Buffett argues, we need to "shatter our current structures . . . that have turned the world into one vast market," one possible strategy would be to reorient economic policy around the aim of full employment and the universal access to education it requires.

While Plato limits justice to the domestic state and foresees no end to tribalism and the inevitability of conflicts among states that vie over territory and wealth, Roosevelt understands domestic justice and security to depend on a new international order. The "cooperation of free countries" will be required to secure domestic freedom, including freedom from want. Roosevelt seeks international collaborations around policies aimed at ensuring full employment globally: "economic understandings which will insure to every nation a healthy peacetime life for its inhabitants—everywhere in the world." Capital ought not to be able to exploit poverty or to take advantage of social inequity, neither nationally nor transnationally.

Roosevelt proves significantly more generous than Rousseau in delineating injustice. Certainly, no one should be so poor, nor social inequity so great, as to find themselves compelled to sell their bodies or body parts, as surrogates, for example, or in an organ market or as a sex slave. Global institutions, as well as states, ought to make freedom from want and the full employment it requires the first aim of all economic policies. Roosevelt foresees that no state on its own will be able to achieve the justice of full employment. International solidarities will be required to create and secure the conditions under which labor can flourish.

The economic collaborations necessary to ensure full employment depend on peace. Only a "world-wide reduction of armaments" can secure the fourth freedom, freedom from fear, on which the other freedoms of expression and religion and freedom from want depend. In a just state, citizens fear neither poverty nor religious persecution nor any danger in free expression. They fear neither one another nor their government and its institutions. While philosophers from Hobbes to Hegel found the state and civil life on fear, Roosevelt makes freeing its citizens from fear the criterion of justice in the state.

Roosevelt envisions a world in which "no nation will be in a position to commit an act of physical aggression against any neighbor." What he does not foresee is the degree to which the state and its economy would become hostage, as Eisenhower warned, to the "military-industrial complex."[28] While discussions of contemporary economic crises regularly focus on the way in which debt is driven by unaffordable benefits accorded to labor, it is worth noting, for example, that for decades in the United States over 20 percent of the annual discretionary budget has been committed to the military and war industry.[29] Without robust international collaborations to ensure global employment, economic disparities will produce global violence. Without a secure peace and global disarmament, the next tyrant only waits for his tactical advantage.

HAPPINESS OR MEANINGFUL WORK: THE POLITICS OF COLLABORATION

Happiness lies not in the mere possession of money; it lies in the joy of achievement, in the thrill of creative effort.

—FRANKLIN D. ROOSEVELT, FIRST INAUGURAL ADDRESS (1933)

Roosevelt's strategy for achieving the domestic and international collaborations that he deems necessary to a more generalized prosperity depends not on a confidence in "free markets" but on a respect for labor. In his analysis, the valorization of moneymaking has resulted in an alienation of destiny. Our destiny, as citizens of a free republic seeking a world of free republics, is "not to be ministered to, but to minster to ourselves and to our fellow-men." Both politics and business have been corrupted by "the falsity of material wealth as a standard of success." It leads the politician to substitute his own pride and profit for the welfare of his constituents, while it produces, in banking and business, "the likeness of callous and selfish wrong-doing."[30] Like Plato, Roosevelt sees the focus on profit as inimical to justice, as well as to the health and happiness of labor and to its productive activities and products. "The mad chase of evanescent profits" has dulled and obscured the "joy and moral stimulation of work." Repeatedly, Roosevelt emphasizes the joy of meaningful work as the core of both happiness and justice.

Perhaps only a few professions offer the "thrill of creative effort," but almost all employment can provide the opportunity for the "joy of achievement."[31]

Roosevelt insists that, in a just state, this opportunity for joy in work will be equal for all. To secure this equality of opportunity, the state must ensure that an effective education is available to all citizens. Without this opportunity early in life to discover and develop her talents, the citizen will not be able to deploy them later. When poor children attend schools that are significantly poorer in quality than those attended by wealthier students, social inequity is reinforced. Justice in the state requires the universal availability of a state education to match the best of the private sector. In developed countries, inequities in education are linked to inequities in health and life expectancy as well as economic security. In developing countries, where educational opportunities are limited and girls are often denied education, the future is compromised for the state and its citizens in both health and economic independence. Globally, lack of education makes it impossible for citizens to mind their own business, and it robs them of their opportunity to experience the joy of meaningful work. These citizens are more likely to find themselves working long hours for low wages and few benefits, or no wages or benefits at all, in tasks in which they are given little independence or opportunity for the sort of "achievement" through labor that Roosevelt describes as the life of a citizen in the just state.

To be meaningful, work must be life sustaining. The existence of a class of "working poor," whose minimum wage or part-time jobs do not pay enough to cover basic expenses such as food and housing, is a symptom of the state's injustice. Freedom from want, on which the other freedoms depend, requires not only an adequate wage but also various forms of life support, including health care and a pension. In addition to his general goals of full employment and disarmament, Roosevelt outlines three specific policy goals related to aspects of the "social economy" that need "immediate improvement." First, pensions and unemployment insurance should be expanded. Second, access to adequate medical care should be expanded. Third, the state needs to devise "a better system by which persons deserving or needing gainful employment may obtain it." Meaningful work not only provides the quotidian needs of life, it also secures the worker against sickness, unemployment, and old age. These policy goals were urgent on January 6, 1941. Without these infrastructures in place, citizens are doomed to live in constant fear of economic ruin, through an illness or protracted unemployment or a penurious retirement. It is urgent that every state act in ways to address these fears, as fear is an invitation to tyranny.

To be meaningful, work must be worth doing and experienced as such by the worker and her community. Meaningful work answers a real need and produces real value in the world of experience. A mother nursing her infant has no doubt that the work is meaningful. A surgeon saving a life has no doubt that her work is meaningful. Garbage collection may not be glamorous, but those who do it know, as firefighters and police do, how essential their labor is to the safety and security of their city.

Telemarketing jobs focused on conning people into buying things they neither want nor need are not meaningful because they are only concerned with profit. Real estate deals in which shoddily built homes in overbuilt tracts are marketed to gullible consumers are not meaningful because they are only concerned with moneymaking. Forklift operators, moving aluminum around all day between a series of warehouses because it allows Goldman Sachs to accrue massive storage fees, know that the work is not meaningful.[32]

To be meaningful, work must be visible and recognized as meaningful by the community. The invisible garment workers in Bangladesh do not enjoy meaningful work. The lack of respect for their labor is painfully illustrated when a catastrophic factory fire occurs or one of the shoddily built factories collapses. Thousands die, yet the Bangladeshi garment industry continues to thrive because the invisible exploitation of this labor is central to the global fashion industry, part of its business model. By reducing actual human beings to an abstract class, decision makers turn their real interests and suffering into an economic calculation of profit and loss. These actual human beings become the object of policies they have no hand in formulating that aim at maximizing their contribution and minimizing their cost to macroeconomic outputs. The abstract name of the population, "Bangladeshi garment workers," insulates consumers against the actual toll in human lives, lives no less passionate and full of hope than the consumers' own.

Similarly, the labor of small farmers, who depend on the informal economy, remains invisible to the metrics of the global economy, making the small farmer vulnerable to the expansionist policies of global agribusiness. If small, indigenous farming can be represented as "unproductive" in global policy discussions, as it often is, then the expansion of agribusiness can be represented as good for the country under "development."[33] This lack of respect for the knowledge and productive labor of indigenous farmers permits agribusiness and policy makers to discount them, and these farmers have little, if any, role in the decisions that affect them. Because global agents fail to recognize and respect their knowledge and expertise, the very way of life of these farmers is threatened, as their lands are turned over to agribusiness or development. Respect for the knowledge accrued over millennia by indigenous farmers ought to be a first principle of global agricultural policy. Justice requires respect for all the labor on which the community depends, from the mundanities of cleaning and washing to the glamours of science and art. In a just state, each citizen contributes in her own way, and all labor deserves respect. Significant social and economic inequity erodes this respect and promotes factionalism and fear.

Finally, to be meaningful, work must not be demeaning. Work can be demeaning because the labor itself is demeaning, as in sex work or some forms of surrogacy. Or it can be demeaning because the boss is demeaning, as in individual cases of sexual harassment or racial discrimination.[34] Beyond these particular instances, workers are often demeaned by the structural forces of sexism and racism. Structural sexism can be at work in individual relationships and in individual judicial cases. For example, a dentist in the United States fired his hygienist based on the claim that her beauty was so great a temptation that it posed a threat to his marriage. He survived judicial scrutiny on the ground that the hygienist was fired not because of her sex but because of her appearance. The court ignored the structure of sexism that operates here, in which women are injured because men find them a temptation.[35] It ignored the injury to the dental assistant not only in economic terms but in terms of the loss of what Roosevelt identified as the condition of happiness, her "joy in achievement." She repeatedly described her loss by saying, "I loved my job." If this man can fire her because of her appearance, then every male dentist is permitted to make hiring decisions on this basis. Indeed, any male employer could fire any female employee on this basis, as the temptation is hardly unique to dentists.

Structural sexism may also create environments in which whole classes or groups of women are demeaned. Female agricultural workers are especially vulnerable given the circumstances of their work, which often involves remote settings with little, if any, oversight or protection. This vulnerability may be compounded for the many immigrants and undocumented workers in agriculture. Women in agriculture are so regularly subject to sexual harassment and rape that these experiences have become structural features of employment.[36] The meaningful work required by the just state is inconsistent with this demeaning devaluation of the worker.

Policy in the just state aims at securing meaningful work for all citizens. First and foremost, educational institutions must be established to give every citizen equal access to the opportunity to discover and develop her talents. The educational infrastructure of the just state provides a culture of possibilities in which each citizen can grow. Inequities in education perpetuate and exacerbate existing social inequities.[37]

Meaningful work is visible and recognized by the community. In the just state, labor elicits the respect of being seen in the mode of looking back, each one acknowledging the work of the other. Meaningful work is worth doing, as it answers to a real need and produces real value. No one is demeaned by meaningful work.

Collaborating internationally to secure full employment, states can create a way of life without an infrastructure of fear. The right to life implies life in a secure landscape free from the fear of violence. It implies economic and social security, as well as physical security, so that a citizen need not be afraid of sickness or old age. Liberty implies the mobility of ideas, speech, and goods, so that each one may enjoy the fruits of her labor in exchange and collaboration with others. The innovation and invention on which prosperity and happiness depend flourish only in a culture where ideas and expressions circulate freely. The right to pursue happiness implies the opportunity (not) to be who I am. It requires an educational infrastructure sufficient to facilitate each one in identifying and developing her talent and passion. At the same time, the educational opportunities must be sufficient to overcome the probabilities that would doom the individual to a life of poverty, fear, and violence.[38] This is the world of meaningful work.

LOOKING BACK AT WOMEN'S LABOR

Unfortunately, Roosevelt does not address "the problem of our time."[39] Whatever his support for women's rights, he assumes the domesticity of women, whose labor has been and remains invisible in the official economy. These women don't "go to work." When they do, the gender division of labor is disturbed in ways that produce significant social crises, from "latchkey children" to an obesity crisis linked to the lack of home cooking. The question keeps recurring: who will feed and care for the children, the sick, and the elderly if women abandon their traditional unpaid and unrecognized labor as family caregivers? Families become dependent on fast food, day-care centers, and nursing homes. Women's work is being commodified through the expansion of low-wage employment in "service" or "caring" professions like health aide or teacher's assistant. Of course, the women in these positions also have families who may not have access to these services and who also need to be cared for. The United States regularly solves its shortage of nurses by recruiting from the Philippines, without wondering about the families that these women have left behind. Instead of enjoying the presence of their mother, the nurse's children receive money, the remittance she sends home every month. Professional women regularly solve the problem of childcare by hiring women of color, who are often undocumented, but these women also have children, and what provision is made for them?

Not only labor but virtually every human institution has been organized around this distinction between the public world of work and the private world of the family; yet no adequate infrastructures exist to support the integration of the two. For millennia, it was assumed that women would remain in the domestic sphere. When women moved into the world of work in significant numbers, they continued, and still continue, to perform the care labor essential to the family.[40] In the United States, unlike many European countries, virtually no supports exist for working mothers, making pregnancy very difficult for working-class mothers. Maternity leave is minimal and rare, even for professional women. Medical care for pregnancy and childbirth is exorbitantly expensive and erratically priced, and women working in low- and medium-wage jobs rarely have adequate insurance.[41] Mothers regularly experience extreme stress over money and incur significant debt. Workplaces rarely supply childcare. Parental leave is, more or less, difficult to take. There are no financial supports for working mothers of young children to rely on other than piecemeal programs for food and housing aimed at the extremely poor.

In France, where the financial supports for motherhood are generous, working women experience a different problem. Once they have children, there is significant social pressure for them to stay home, and the transition back to the workplace is difficult.[42] Despite state support for the family, women in France remain underrepresented in the councils that determine the future. They hold about the same percentage of leadership positions in politics, business, and academia as their American counterparts.[43]

Similarly, professional women in the United States, who enjoy educational and economic privilege, also experience the lack of adequate infrastructures for integrating work and family. In the last decade, a wave of professional women has attested to the difficulties they face in dividing their time and energy between the two. A recent survey of Ivy League graduates revealed a trend among these women toward domesticity and away from work in the public sphere. They repeatedly cited the suffering they had witnessed in their mothers as they attempted to achieve at work while striving to care for their families.[44] The suffering of these working mothers, significant enough to turn their daughters away from work, is a symptom of the urgent need for new infrastructures to sustain both work and family.

Our time calls for concepts that "shatter our current structures," not only by reconfiguring economic relations but also by reimagining the infrastructures of space and time to facilitate women's generativity as mothers and workers. How might the built environment be reconstructed, and daily schedules revised, to support women's labor in all its domains of employment? Until these questions become the focus of policy debates, the state will suffer from the loss of women's labor in the public sphere and from the damage to both work and family that results from the antagonism between the two.

In many parts of the world, of course, women face far more difficult situations and choices than those of professional women in the West. They are often treated as property and married at a very young age without consultation. They begin their lives of labor so young as to almost miss having a childhood. Often denied education, these women are deprived of the skills and ideas that might enable them to imagine a future of meaningful work.

On a visit to Rajasthan in 2010, I was struck by how hard the women worked. At dawn, they climb steep hills to collect firewood. By noon, they descend in groups of eight or ten, each one carrying an enormous bundle of sticks and limbs on her head, usually larger than the girl or woman herself. Several times during the day, they haul the family's water from the local well. At other times, the women are cooking or sweeping the house. They seem to be always working, while the men of the village occasionally work in their shops, but are to be found more often drinking chai. A young woman of thirty-five looks fifty after more than two decades of daily, continuous, hard labor and several children.[45]

In a remote corner of Rajasthan, however, I discovered women engaged in a collaboration that transgressed the gender division of labor and provided a culture of meaningful work and joy. As I approached Dastkari Kendra in Ranthambore, I realized that it was the first time in India that I had encountered women laughing. From some distance, I could hear several dozen women of all ages chattering and laughing with unrestrained joy. The women sat in their splendid saris, bright orange, acid green, cherry red, on the floor of an open porch. Each one had busy hands. One group was making a patchwork quilt. Another was making fans. Several women were drawing designs for block printing. Not far away was a group of potters working at their wheels. And just inside, off the porch, women were tie-dyeing and block-printing fabrics out of which they would make clothes in both Western and Indian styles, table linens, and purses. The Dastkar Craft Community Center provides employment for women and men from agrarian villages that were displaced by the Ranthambore Tiger Park. The land onto which they were relocated could not sustain an agrarian economy, and the Ranthambore Foundation asked Dastkar Society for Crafts and Craftspeople to work with the villagers to create a viable economy in crafts and handiwork.

Not only have the villagers created a thriving economy, Dastkari Kendra has changed their lives by introducing them to the joyful collaborations of meaningful work. The women were suspicious at first, and the Dastkar Society organizers understood that its task was to help them "discover their hidden potential."[46] By sending its craftspeople to live in the villages and work with the villagers, Dastkar gained their trust, and, within six months, more than seventy-five women were participating. Twenty-five years later, more than three hundred craftspeople participate. Dastkari Kendra has changed the villagers' attitudes toward caste, purdah, marriage, and religion. Initially, they segregated themselves according to caste or religion, but their joyful collaboration has created a democratic space where people mingle freely across these distinctions. The economic independence of the women has not only improved their material quality of life, and that of their children, it has also reshaped gender relations in the villages, with women taking leadership roles both in the craft collective and in other local institutions. The collective demonstrates how the happy collaborations of meaningful work can overcome inequity and the violence of racism and sexism.

Dastkar quotes the local doctor: "I can recognize a Dastkar craftswoman from half a kilometer away, just by the way she walks and holds her head." Unlike the disrobing gaze of Rousseau's governor or the lascivious eye of Zeus, the doctor looks back at a humanbody that commands respect. These women have found the meaningful work on which, as Roosevelt argued, health and happiness as well as the peace of the community depend. They have found the "joy of achievement" along with economic independence and social recognition.

Justice is neither an illusion nor a dream. It is an achievable reality of which material examples currently exist.[47]

States and global actors need to "try out concepts that shatter our current structures." Most important, states need to address inequities in education that perpetuate inequities in life and to insure that everyone has the opportunity to experience the "joy of achievement" in meaningful work. These philosophical commitments have clear implications for public policy, if the latter can be freed from the myths and rhetoric as well as the interests of globalization. States might begin by making full employment and equity in education the standard of economic and political success.

Roosevelt imagined a world in which citizens of every state are unafraid and free to think and speak and worship or not as they will. He understood that the confusion of state power and religion produces factionalism and violence. He knew that the vitality of innovation and invention on which economic success depends only grows in a culture of free and unfettered expression. He aimed to lead the United States and other nations toward a world in which no one lives in fear of violence and in which sickness and old age are not haunted by fear of economic ruin. Perhaps he did not fully appreciate the need to address the gender division of labor as an impediment to full employment and happiness for women and men, but his narrative offers a counterforce to capital's rhetoric of globalization, and, in a time of chatter, ineptitude, and self-interest, he stands up for the right, for a world in which each one is sustained in the collaborative project of finding and pursuing meaningful work.

PART FOUR
Sovereign Bodies
POLITICS OF WONDER OR
THE RIGHT TO BE JOYFUL

Because of who my father is, I've been able to occupy some seats I never expected to sit in. Inside any important philanthropy meeting, you witness heads of state meeting with investment managers and corporate leaders. All are searching for answers with their right hand to problems that the others in the room have created with their left. . . . As more lives and communities are destroyed by the system that creates vast amounts of wealth for the few, the more heroic it sounds to "give back." . . . But this just keeps the existing structure of inequity in place. . . . Money should be spent trying out concepts that shatter our current structures and systems that have turned much of the world into one vast market. Is progress really Wi-Fi on every corner? No. It's when no 13-year-old girl on the planet gets sold for sex. But as long as most folks pat themselves on the back for charitable acts, we've got a perpetual poverty machine.

—PETER BUFFETT, "THE CHARITABLE-INDUSTRIAL COMPLEX" (2013)

We all have to breathe, feed, clothe, and house ourselves. Our societies are controlled by this need, which rightful as it is, accords money a power that its totally disproportionate—a power rarely questioned by democratic regimes even though it inevitably leads to new hierarchies between rich and poor and between affluent and impoverished countries, along with a redistribution system based upon pity and upon appeals to share, which potentially exacerbate loss of human dignity and authoritarian relations between people.

Of course, sharing is better than leaving someone to die of starvation. But this always involves the power of some over others, a power mediated by money . . . in money humanity has alienated its freedom and its culture.

—LUCE IRIGARAY, *I LOVE TO YOU* (1996)

There is a sense of wonder, and mystery, vouchsafed in the wave of happiness and laughter emerging from the foul and squalid tenements of the poor. It is not a question of innocence contrasted with experience, because these children were not innocent, but somehow a triumph of the human imagination over the city. Even in the midst of filth, they have the need and the right to be joyful.

—PETER ACKROYD, *LONDON: A BIOGRAPHY* (2012)

BEGINNING FROM HUMANBODIES, an ethics of life effects a transformation in the philosophical concept of the universal, for it is no longer possible in philosophy to think truth under the figure of the One. The fiction of the one subject Man and his rights may have run its course, but the universality of women's experiences has only just begun to be thought. Only the hubris that permeates the concept of Man could lead to the conclusion that its exhaustion constitutes the end of history. If history is, as Hegel argues, the story of the slave regaining his freedom, there is still a great deal more to come, and not only in the masculine voice.[1]

The ironic universality of humanbodies is that every body occurs as a specificity: this one. "*Once* to everything, only *once*. *Once* and no more. And we too, *once*. And never again."[2] What is universal in the experience of humanbodies is just this specificity and identity of the body. You—*you*—are not just an instance of a general form. Human experience only occurs in the first person. The material immediacy and determination of each humanbody as a unique "once" is irreparable and cannot be reduced to an abstract form or name, figures that are logically inappropriate to it. As in Hobbes, abstraction is always allied to mastery. The use of general forms and abstract names to facilitate and sustain the disposition of populations constitutes prima facie ethical harm.[3] This is particularly true in medicine when the specificity of the patient is lost in the case or protocol.[4]

As these specific and irreplaceable bodies, we find ourselves always already connected by our generation and generativity to other humanbodies. Our bodies belong to a certain history and place and are constituted by its climates and verdures, its landscapes and habits. Every humanbody lives in a specific culture of possibilities that sustains specific forms of life. The others, differentiated and always sexed, are not reducible to "the Other," a concept that belongs to philosophy's logic of the same, nor to "the brother" of property's fraternal logic.[5] Others are always differentiated and sexed, and the male has had his turn as the paradigm.

At the same time, every humanbody needs to live in a sustainable relation with Earth and the elements, for the humanbody is truly of the fertile soil, *humus,* not some supersensible realm. Each of us, each humanbody, me and you too, needs light and air, the heat of the sun, clean water. Each of us gets hungry and needs to eat. Each of us needs a way to get rid of our wastes without being poisoned by them. These needs, though articulated with the specificity of humanbodies themselves, constitute our universal human condition.

To prosper, each humanbody needs to enjoy the integrity of its specificity, rather than be reduced to an abstract name or disposed of through a general image. To thrive as an agent, each one must enjoy the integrity of her body, including her generativity. Generativity, genuine agency or creativity as a mode of life, grows in the safety of the nonviolent place; in a sustainable relation to the elements of Earth and human needs; and in the mobility of humanbodies, ideas, and things that freedom from fear makes possible.

For millennia, philosophical definitions of human being installed, as if forever, a bifurcated self, one half embodied and material, the other hypothetical and speculative.[6] For at least three and a half centuries, this unhappy consciousness has based the forms of life on a fear of death and on the violence engendered by that fear, as if the violence necessary to the security of property and sexual propriety were a fact of nature, as if the law of property and the social inequity it legitimated were inevitable, as if the market that serves the increasing concentration, rather than circulation, of wealth and power were imposed by an alien and absolute power.

In our time, the lines of force deployed upon humanbodies through Man's codes, forms, abstract names, institutions, practices, policies, and procedures comprise a field as vast and complex as the physical forces of nature. Critical phenomenology, however, makes the familiar strange and exposes the nonnecessity of Man. Is it possible any longer to believe in the mythology of the originary violence, in the necessity of property and sexual propriety, in the divine right of capital, in the rights of wealth, and, for the rest, compensations from the beyond? Even Hegel understood that the law of property is no more logically coherent or required than the idea of ownership in common.[7] Critical phenomenology exposes these tropes as contingent historical formations. We might have begun elsewhere.

We might begin again elsewhere, from the engendering of each and all in the body of a woman. In our time it seems as if a misguided respect for "cultural differences" must preclude certain kinds of solidarity, indeed any solidarity that would claim to be universal. At the same time, in many international contexts where "human rights" are at issue, "cultural difference" serves as a cheap argument for maintaining untouched systems of subjection that are deployed upon living humanbodies, depriving them of their agency and integrity.[8] A culture that treats women as property, whether in Saudi Arabia or the U.S. National Football League, does not deserve respect.[9] Remembering that each and every one has been born of a woman opens up new possibilities of solidarity. This thought installs each and every one as a historical, relational, and generational being, always already interdependent with other living beings amidst the improbable and wondrous profusion of life on Earth.

Nothing is more vulnerable than the infant humanbody that we all have been, which is universal in us. Without mobility or speech, unable to feed herself, cold, helpless: this is where it all began. The mother takes up the infant and puts her to her breast: for thousands of years, women have been generating society in this simple gesture.

I will bear this child.

Man's hegemony began with the power to name and the elaboration of the signs of power as the virtual dimension of an immanent violence. When Man named woman, he made her his property, a weak appendage without agency, but also his conscience and his muse and the fertile body of his generation. Absolutely dependent, but also, as Rousseau insists, absolutely responsible for his happiness, she is the mother of all ironies.

Under the regime of the rights of Man, sovereignty constitutes an instituted power over a corporate body. The sovereign power or "Artificiall Person" acts as the head to the corporate body politic comprised, as in Hobbes' frontispiece, of the actual bodies of subjects who provide the hands and feet of his agency. Under this sovereign power, an individual human body cannot enjoy its own integrity and specificity; rather, it exists only as a member of the body politic, more or less ensanguinated or necrotic.

Critical phenomenology rethinks sovereignty as natural and dispersed in individual bodies. Each one should enjoy a sustainable relation to bodily needs and have the opportunity to thrive in meaningful work. Each one should enjoy the free mobility of ideas, images, words, and things. Political mobility implies negotiation, forgiveness, and moving forward instead of clinging hardheadedly and hardheartedly to the debts and resentments that generate factionalism and tribal violence, whether those tribes are religious, cultural, racial, or political. Each one should be able to pursue happiness and to live free of fear, free from both fear of want and fear of violence.

While social contract theory and Man's human rights regimes focus on the bearer of rights who makes a claim for himself and must defend his rights, critical phenomenology bases ethics and politics on being *claimed by the right*. Like Antigone, we find ourselves under obligations installed by the continuity of generations and the possibilities of our own generativity. No one should be so poor as to need to sell herself for sex or to sell her organs or to sell her daughter in marriage, and no one should be so rich as to be able to afford to buy another's body, nor should anyone make profit from the use of another body and its generativity.[10] No thirteen-year-old girl should be sold for sex anywhere on the planet. No fifteen-year-old boy should have a gun thrust into his hands and be urged to kill anywhere on the planet. No one should be murdered for marrying according to her will anywhere on the planet. No girl should be shot for going to school anywhere on the planet. These are universal truths that call for transnational solidarities. They claim us as the right.

Like every man, each woman is sovereign in her own body, yet her sovereignty cannot be reduced to his. While a man reproduces in the body of another, a woman reproduces in her own body.[11] Her natural sovereignty includes sovereignty over this distinctive generativity, yet this natural sovereignty remains politically insecure or unsecured. In arrogating to themselves authority over a woman's generativity, the church and the state are guilty of *pleonexia* or injustice. They claim for themselves decisions that belong to her, as if they could preempt her, representing her as a body with no agency or interiority of its own, a body to be acted upon, not acting for itself. Until women are sovereign in determining their own reproductive destinies, until they are free from the "tutelage of the Church and the State," they remain less than citizens. They are cast as a population that "cannot be trusted with these decisions."[12] Religious arguments that pit a fertilized egg or embryo or fetus against the agency and citizenship of women have no place in political philosophy or in democratic politics. Philosophy and politics must eschew not only the abstractions essential to science but also the speculations of religious faith. It is past time for the state and the church to "mind their own business," as justice requires.[13] It is past time for them to start trusting women, leaving women's decisions to women. It is past time for the church and the state to start paying attention to their own business, to their obligations to create political infrastructures that respect women's sovereignty and material infrastructures that sustain women's generativity.

Recent data demonstrate how common an unplanned pregnancy is, even when women responsibly practice birth control.[14] Nearly one out of every three women will experience an unplanned pregnancy at some point in her life. Treating an unwanted pregnancy requires uncomplicated medical intervention that should be readily accessible without restriction as part of basic health care.[15] The current sequestering of these services in the United States, separating their delivery from the rest of health care, is not morally sustainable and exposes women and their caregivers to both hardship and violence.[16] There should be no more debate about these medical services than any other, and they should be fully integrated into medical education and the delivery of medical care.

Women's bodies incorporate a hollow or fold that can expand to provide a necessary place for another human being, from conception to infancy. And, so far, every human being in history has entered the world through the body of a woman. Theories of intersubjectivity are unnecessary to establish the relation to others as constitutive of each individual's identity: women's bodies and the history of every humanbody already demonstrate conclusively the presence of the other in each one, the dependence of each one on an other. Women's bodies provide the portal by which each and every one joins the species of other humanbodies. Let us begin here with the moral relationships inscribed in our own bodies. The right to life begins when a woman says, "I will bear this child."

Beginning here does not imply any obligation on the part of a particular woman to bear a child. This imposes on women no obligation to mother; rather, it installs, for each and all, *the right to have been mothered*. Let every infant come into a world welcomed by a mother who is supported as an agent in her own right. Let each child come into a world where her mother is not afraid of violence or poverty. Let each child come into a world where her mother is confident her children will enjoy a culture of possibilities that promotes their agency and generativity. Let the church and the state mind their business of securing for every mother and her child freedom from fear and want and the confidence in a future of meaningful work. Critical phenomenology valorizes mother and child as a privileged point of political intervention, not an image of any particular woman's destiny.[17]

Mothering, like some other forms of care, has as its aim letting the other go free. Each of us depended on the generativity of mothers. Each of us depended on the generosity of the others, who, instead of trying to own and contain us, worked to let us go free, free to enjoy the sovereignty of our own bodies. The agency of the generative mother who cultivates the difference of her child from herself provides a model for human relationships. Against philosophy's narrative of the encounter with the other as a scene of threat, violence, and fear, critical phenomenology reveals others as surprising and excessive. Against the account of politics as a relation to others figured as the same, critical phenomenology locates ethical thinking in the "advent" of the other who cannot be anticipated.[18] Taking seriously the irreducibility of the other introduces into experience a wild novelty that cannot be tamed by reason and that commands respect. "There is something passionate, generous, and sacred in us which exceeds the representations of the mind: it is this excess which makes us human."[19] Resisting the habitual impulse to reduce the other to the same, to relate to others through property and privilege, or to determine her worth as a "Price" set in the market, wondering before the other provides a "bridge to the future."[20] The time of wondering before the other belongs neither to the mythic time outside history nor to the historical chronology of Man's regime of rights and his triumph over (his) nature. "The problem of *we* is that of a meeting which occurs through fortune, good fortune, (a *kairos*?) ... but it is also or especially that of a constituting temporality: together, with, between."[21] *Kairos* names an opportunity, an opening, a chance that appears between, that humanbodies enjoy together.

FROM SOVEREIGNTY TO SOLIDARITY

Wondering before the other opens up the possibility of a new ethics of the imagination focused on reimagining the infrastructures of life to promote not only human health and happiness but also the flourishing of Earth and other living creatures. Ethics and politics should focus, not on property, sexual propriety, or ascribing blame and praise, but on "what is to be done and how to do what is necessary to guarantee the existence of a world that is livable in the future."[22] Like Peter Buffett, Irigaray and Foucault call for "shattering our current structures." It is the task of philosophy not only to reflect on the disasters that threaten existence and Earth but also to create a new culture of possibilities that would "convert individual morality into collective ethics."[23] Philosophers must unite politics and happiness by "refusing to accept that politics should be reduced to managing a world that is now dehumanized and dehumanizing; by refusing to accept that the world should remain as it is."[24] While some might "hanker after a little monarchy in the world of ideas,"[25] philosophy requires "a certain determination to throw off familiar ways of thought and to look at the same things in a different way; a passion for seizing what is happening now and what is disappearing; a lack of respect for the traditional hierarchies of what is important and fundamental."[26] Foucault warns against the tendency to turn wonder before the other and genealogical critique into a "political program."[27] Yet he always writes with a political intent, intervening disruptively just where the subject has been subjected to provide him with the chance *not* to become who he is, that is, who he is destined to be by the current logic of fraternity and capital.

Both Foucault and Irigaray valorize curiosity as the distinctively philosophical attitude. The philosopher does not know what to expect, but is open to the advent of the unexpected and unpredictable others. The task of philosophy, of ethics and politics, is to generate solidarities that sustain the sovereignty of each differentiated human body. Collaborative projects infused with the hope of a new future build solidarities, while according to each one his or her own share of responsibility. Working together toward freedom from fear and want might begin to "create bridges between today and tomorrow."

Justice requires the encouragement of a form of economic development that is appropriate to the environment and specific to the culture of a country. It requires the promotion of "economic diversity rather than imposing a single and inevitably competitive model."[28] In our time, macroeconomic actors like the World Bank, the International Monetary Fund, and global corporations, particularly agribusiness and the oil and war industries, overshadow or dwarf the agency of democratic states, usurping their power to represent and serve their citizens adequately. Until this "current structure" is "shattered," extreme wealth will continue to assuage its conscience with philanthropy to solve problems it has itself created. In the industrialized world these structures have produced an "austerity" politics that demonizes collaborations around public welfare while significantly increasing social, economic, and political inequity. Attempts to impose these structures in the "developing" world disrupt rural economies, displace investment in local infrastructures, and regularly result in the forced migration of peoples from rural to urban areas, with all the attendant ills of poverty and social alienation.

The "hidden roots" of nationalism, conflict, and war lie in "the refusal to question and change one's own habits."[29] Health and happiness require that the interest of living together on Earth trump Man's honor and property. War is not "grafted upon human nature,"[30] nor is it "indispensable to the perfectibility of human cultures."[31] War results from Man's "unsociability" and his valorization of his own honor and property over life. It is past time for Man's reeducation. The idea that conflicts can be addressed by arming the "right" faction or by introducing more war machinery into a culture is ludicrous, and, if we are to survive, this familiar idea must become strange. War creates brutality and feeds cycles of revenge. Sometimes it may be necessary for a people to defend itself against aggression, but, historically and today, war has served privilege, wealth, and those who profit from the war industry.

The conditions of work need to be restructured, not only to overcome the gender division of labor on which the modern nation-state is based and to allow for the integration of work and family, but also to elevate generativity, nourishing and sustaining the agency of others, as an essential form of labor, as valuable a form of labor as any a human can undertake. It is time for philosophy to stop theorizing identity based on property and sex. It is time to bring the former to justice, which will require not philanthropy but "shattering our current structures," and time to let the latter proliferate on its own.[32] It is time for philosophy and the state to take collaboration and meaningful work as the locus of identity. It is past time for the state to recognize full employment as essential to justice and the criterion of a just state. It is past time for an economic restructuring that rewards the work of educating and caring for others, rather than the gambling in financial markets that serves only a privileged few and furthers the concentration of wealth in their hands.

The sustaining Earth and its elements, as well as its biodiversity, command respect, not only because human life depends on them, but also because, like the others, nature has the power to invoke the wonder and awe that prevent humanbodies from becoming mere calculators of interest. "Wildlife is and should be useless in the same way art, music, poetry, and even sports are useless. They are useless in the sense that they do nothing more than raise our spirits, make us laugh or cry, frighten, disturb, and delight us. They connect us not just to what's weird, different, other, but to a world where we humans do not matter nearly as much as we like to think. And that should be enough."[33] The spider *mastophora dizzy-deani* "fling[s] a ball of silk on a thread like a spitball to snag moths out of the air." Its name honors both its own wonderful mode of life and the life of one of the greatest baseball players of all time. Dizzy Dean was known not only for his superior pitching but also for his antics and his creativity. "When ole Diz was out there pitching it was more than just another ball game. It was a regular three-ring circus and everybody was wide awake and enjoying being alive."[34] Gratitude for Dean's unique style of play informs the name of the spider whose style reminded the scientist of the pitcher's originality and panache. And we can enjoy not only the style of Dean and the spider but also the creativity and sense of humor in the scientist who associated them.

It is past time for humanity to dispense with Man's idea that nature is his to master and a resource to be plundered. It is past time for humanity to valorize wonder over need in relation to nature. Human exceptionalism arises not from Man's ability to reason—as Hobbes argued, animals deliberate too—but from the fact that human existence is not determined by the *differentiae* of the species. Unlike other animals, whose tooth or claw, haunch or hearing, determine them as predator and prey, humans must choose how to eat and how to live. Human exceptionalism does not imply mastery over nature but a responsibility to sustain nature and biodiversity for the next generation.[35] Nature's biodiversity claims us to tend it, because we alone among all creatures can. Human exceptionalism consists not in the ability to subdue nature to rational utility but in being claimed by the right.

Resentment and despair, greed and jealousy, hatred and the spirit of revenge will undermine collective efforts to "shatter our current structures," but that only makes collaboration all the more urgent and necessary. These collaborations themselves build solidarity, which does not preexist them in some common property. Solidarity arises in and out of the irreducible difference of the other. Nadine Gordimer had little in common with Nelson Mandela, but together they struggled and won a measure of justice for their nation. Fannie Lou Hammer had little in common with white college students, but she inspired them to join her cause and built a coalition that made a difference as the tide of civil rights moved across the South. Everyone wants to enjoy the right to life or freedom from fear and want. Everyone wants to enjoy liberty or the free mobility of person, words, ideas, and goods. Everyone wants the opportunity to pursue happiness through education and meaningful work. The aim of a livable future calls for collaborations that can produce new solidarities based neither on the fiction of a generic subject nor on the politics of identity.

Bodies proliferate under global capital: the models and professional cheerleaders who sell their sex for low pay in a dangerous and short career; the highschool girls subjected to dress codes that teach them to fear their sexuality and to believe that men's violence against women is something they themselves have provoked; the girls at play who must be taught, Rousseau insists, that they have no right to be at liberty; the Gilgo girls driven by underemployment to sex work and murdered; the surrogate or organ supplier who is so poor that she sees no choice but to sell her own body to someone rich enough to buy it.

But other incandescent bodies exceed the calculus of profit and loss and transgress sexual propriety. The beautiful young girls, as refreshing as a draught of cold water on a hot day, still play together joyfully in a meadow of flowers, reflected in the eye of their leader. The mother would not abandon her daughter. The two mothers guard the fecundity of Earth and the wild profusion of life. The mother spoke up and spoke out against her daughter's shaming by a school dress code. The girls of Morris Knolls High spoke up for themselves against the codes' complicity with a culture of rape. The Dastkar women enjoy meaningful work, and their joy infuses the way they walk and carry themselves in their community. The girl with a book will not be scared away from school, even by extreme violence. These women, vulnerable, marginalized, prove resilient enough to be the locus of generativity and the keepers of the seed: the water bearer, herder of ducks and geese, the milkmaid, poultry farmer, gardener, gatherer, cook, teacher, and nurse. For millennia women have fed their families, raised their children, and buried their dead.

This labor commands respect, and all humanbodies are responsible for it. Women are no more determined by their *differentiae* than men. Only under the gender division of labor and the right to property is it possible to read a woman's destiny in her body. Only if the state or the church denies women access to basic health care does she lack the means to manage her reproductive destiny. A girl with a book, freed from the gender division of labor, poses just as much of a risk and a question as her brother. She too enjoys the right (not) to become who she is. Justice requires not only that "no 13-year-old girl on the planet gets sold for sex," but also that every 13-year-old girl on the planet, and every boy too, have the opportunity to answer the question of her being with the full plasticity of her brain, hands, and feet. Her generativity may take many forms, including motherhood, but no prejudice can be sustained that would determine her destiny in advance. Surprising, novel, unheard-of identities can be expected.

Once and never again.

"But this *once* to have been, if only this *once*: to have been of the earth seems beyond revoking."

◆ ◆ ◆ ◆

The whale resurfaces. The humans huddled on deck in the wind and spray, puny by comparison to the great leviathan, release cries of awe and joy at its mighty grace. Together, they have traveled far, and they find themselves bound to each other by a wonder that leaves to nature its uselessness. The whale dives, having answered their need and right to be joyful.

Thank you, dear reader, for your collaboration, for your time and mind and heart, for coming along with me from sovereignty to solidarity.

Notes

1. In 2011 King Abdullah decreed that Saudi women would have the right to vote and run for municipal office. The activation of the right was delayed until 2015. The decree did not address the myriad practical difficulties in exercising such rights for citizens who cannot drive, who cannot go out in public or travel on their own, and who have no financial independence. In late 2014 the Saudi government has undertaken a campaign to solve the obstacles to women's participation in the labor force. A major obstacle is mobility, as women can neither drive nor take public transportation.

2. Despite the persistence of virulent racism in the U.S. and the slow pace of change in South Africa, the cultures of Jim Crow and apartheid have ceased to exist, and black Americans and South Africans enjoy greater, if still unequal, mobility and opportunity. The demise of these cultures required not only the extraordinary courage and solidarity of the oppressed but also political solidarities across racial lines. Attempts at transcultural critique around gender are frequently charged with a lack of respect for indigenous values. If those "values," however, impose the systematic subjection of a class of people, is critique not warranted? Justice requires this transcultural critique to open up channels of solidarity and generate the kind of individual and collective outrage and action against gender inequity that terminated apartheid and Jim Crow.

   Critics of the cultures of gender inequity are also charged with failing to respect the women of these cultures by denying them agency, which ignores the dependency of agency on a culture of possibilities that respects and sustains it. The aim of the critique is not to impose policies, but to expose structural injustice and foster solidarities. The exposure of gender inequity and the effort to form collaborations outweigh the risk of appearing imperious.

3. In 1995 two male officials decided that the Miami Gulliver Prep School girls cross-country team would be stripped of its third-place finish in a two-mile race at a state meet because their running shorts were too short. The high-cut shorts were being worn by distinguished athletes like Jackie Joyner-Kersee and Gail Devers. Twenty years later, they are ubiquitous. Recently, a wave of dress codes in public middle schools in the western United States has focused on the need to regulate girls' attire in order to prevent boys from being distracted. See the discussion of dress codes in chapter 2.

4. In the 2014 Supreme Court decision Burwell v. Hobby Lobby, despite the opposition of the Court's three distinguished female members, five male justices perverted the law by subordinating women's reproductive freedom to a religious interest. In many states women who seek certain reproductive services, from IUDs to the termination of pregnancy, are subject to restrictions in access, as well as demeaning and intrusive efforts to manipulate or preempt their decision making. In 2011, for example, Texas passed a law requiring all women seeking an abortion to undergo a sonogram, frequently transvaginally. The patient is asked to view the sonogram and to listen to the fetal heartbeat. The law states that the doctor is "required" to display the images of the fetus and make the heartbeat audible. The patient may decline to view the images or listen to the heartbeat, but she must listen to the doctor's explanation of the images and the fetus's development. She must then wait twenty-four hours before having an abortion. The law not only places an undue burden on women's health clinics, it also disrespects women's moral agency and bodily integrity in favor of sectarian religious beliefs.

5. See Irigaray, "The Question of the Other," 132–33.

6. The topic has been a constant for decades in both the popular and scholarly press. See Brody, *Women in the Middle*. For a summary of research themes, see Bianchi and Milke, "Work and Family Research."

7. Hegel, *Elements of the Philosophy of Right*, #166, n. 2.

8. Wolfson and Bleich, "Is Cooking at Home Associated?" See also Nguyan and Powell, "The Impact of Restaurant Consumption." See also Cutler, Glaeser, and Shapiro, "Why Have Americans Become More Obese?" While Cutler and his colleagues dispute the claim that an increase in eating out rather than at home is associated with obesity, they clearly demonstrate the link between obesity and commercially processed or "mass preparation" foods.

9. See Eva Feder Kittay's analysis of the universality of dependency in *Love's Labor*, 29–30.

10. Husserl's phenomenological *epoché*, especially in its transcendental form, assumes that the density of habits and attitudes can be suspended by thinking it so. Critical phenomenology respects the thickness of experience and the immense work, both conceptual and practical, that is required to expose its assumptions and prejudices.

11. Foucault's method is not "transcendental" in that it is not a transcendentalism: it does not seek abstract formal structures but the infrastructures of historically determined ways of saying, thinking, and doing. It does aim at transcending this form of subjectiv-

ity: it aims at "the possibility of no longer being, doing, or thinking what we are, do, or think." *Ethics*, 315–16. The work of philosophy is to "think otherwise, to do something else, to become other than what one is" (327).

12. Foucault, *Ethics*, 315. Critical phenomenology proposes an uneasy marriage between Foucault's genealogical analysis of the infrastructures of experience and Irigaray's account of the implications for thought and life of the irreducibility of sexual difference. Neither Foucault not Irigaray would happily embrace the label *phenomenologist*; however, both undertake a critical project in order to change the conditions of experience to open up a new future. For both, experience is not merely an object of thought, but a vital urgency. Philosophy's task is not merely to think, but to change the possibilities of life by thinking anew.

13. Ibid., 327.

14. A culture is a complex of infrastructures, material and discursive, that supports specific forms of life. The question about culture is "what grows in it?" Beyond this understanding of culture as a medium of life, any theory of culture should be resisted as an attempt to install a general image in place of the irreducibly specific identity of any culture. The truth of any culture is the specificity of what grows in it.

No doubt South Africans still contend with the legacy of apartheid, as U.S. Southerners still negotiate the racism of slavery and Jim Crow, but these political structures no longer exist and no longer provide the conditions of life for these cultural forms.

15. Hobbes, *Leviathan*, chapter 5, p. 35. See also *Elements of Law Natural and Politic*, chapter XV.1.

16. Kittay, "Equality, Dignity and Disability," 110.

17. UNESCO Declaration on Bioethics and Human Rights (2005).

18. UNESCO Bioethics website, May 2014.

19. O'Neill, plenary address, 2008.

20. Turner, "Global Health Inequalities and Bioethics."

21. In France, for example, only heterosexual couples have access to assisted reproduction. In the United States access is significantly limited by wealth.

22. See, e.g., Russell et al., "The Role of Cost-Effectiveness Analysis."

23. On the way in which the unresolved conflict between these equally commanding needs falls differentially on women, see Smith, "Elder Care, Gender, and Work."

24. Foucault, *The Hermeneutics of the Subject*.

25. On the complicity of bioethics and corporate and state actors, see DeBruin, "Ethics on the Inside" and Charo, "The 'Endarkenment.'"

26. See Khader, *Adaptive Preferences and Women's Empowerment*. Khader's analysis of "adaptive preferences" shows how it might be possible to criticize structures of subjection without impugning the remarkable agency of the subjected. Bioethics should serve the creation of solidarities with all the girls and women who, each and every one, have a right to mobility and education.

27. Alison Jaggar is particularly eloquent in her critique of cross-cultural analyses that do not take into account the force of global capital and other geopolitical forces in

shaping women's experience in middle- and low-income countries. See Jaggar, "Global Responsibility and Western Feminism."

INTRODUCTION

1. Baudrillard, *The Agony of Power*, 61.
2. In the 2012 U.S. presidential election, the two parties, the two candidates, and their supporters spent more than $2 billion. The recent Supreme Court decision in Mc-Cutcheon v. Federal Election Commission (October 2013) continues to facilitate the influence of wealth in democratic representation. This recent trend began with Citizen's United v. Federal Election Commission (October 2009) in which, by a five to four vote, the court characterized corporate campaign contributions as free speech protected by the First Amendment. www.supremecourt.gov/opinions/09pdf/08–205 .pdf. In keeping with the thoroughgoing irony of our time, "The system [even, the system of laws] doesn't care a fig for laws, it unleashes deregulation in every domain" (ibid., 49). The law "cannibalizes" itself.
3. For an analysis of the no-place and disposability of place under global capital, see Rawlinson, "Toward an Ethics of Place"; cf. Baudrillard, *The Agony of Power*, 102, on tourism as "terrifying" and "a form of terror."
4. Irigaray makes a similar point. See *Democracy Begins Between Two*, 159:

   > We know what the relationship is between industrialization, capitalism, and slavery. We also know the limits of industrialization with regard to employment, yet we go on involving other countries in this process and, in this way, win a few more years for an economic regime whose blind alleys should be all too obvious to us.
   >
   > In my view, it would be fairer politically-speaking to encourage a form of economic development that was appropriate to the environment and culture of a country, in other words to promote economic diversity rather than imposing a single and inevitably competitive model.

5. Baudrillard gives a more extensive analysis of "whiteness" in *Carnival and Cannibal*.
6. Baudrillard, *The Agony of Power*, 52.
7. Ibid., 106. Baudrillard adduces as evidence the various walls that are constructed to protect the democratic space from the Other: the wall constructed along the U.S./Mexico border or the wall that separates the Israelis from the Palestinians. Whereas the dominated wanted to escape the contained space of the ghetto or Iron Curtain, the discriminated want to get in, to the place of "unlimited growth and prosperity."
8. In his famous Four Freedoms speech (1941), FDR argues that a democratic republic cannot be isolationist, as its continued existence and flourishing depends on transnational solidarities and collaborations: "the cooperation of free countries, working together." Perhaps, it will not be so easy to dismiss this historical referent; FDR anticipates Baudrillard's own critique of wealth, privilege, and violence as forces undermining democratic process even as he poses against them "freedom from fear—which, translated into world terms means a world-wide reduction of armaments. . . . This

is no vision of a distant millennium. It is a definite basis for a kind of world attainable in our own time." Roosevelt, "The 'Four Freedoms' Speech." Perhaps it is only via a historical referent that it is possible to escape irony. Is it no longer possible for an American president to say, at least with a straight face, that he will not allow a "small group of selfish men . . . [to] clip the wings of the American eagle in order to feather their own nests"? (292). Sometimes, the "axis of evil" is real. If it is necessary to dispel the specters of evil unleashed by Bush/Cheney through truth and reconciliation, it is no less necessary to imitate or perform the courage of the imagination that reimagines the world on behalf of life, including a reimagining of the way business is done. This risk of appearing nostalgic, the risk of appearing not to get the bad joke of history becoming parody and farce, hardly provides sufficient reason to cede the discourse of the universal, any more than that of life or solidarity.

9. A certain concept of woman has always operated to sustain Man. Hegel names woman the "eternal irony of the community." Baudrillard was not the first to identify irony as the rhetorical and material horizon of "our time."

10. Hartigan, in *Sin City*.

I: CRITIQUE OF RIGHTS

1. Hobbes, *Leviathan*, chapter 17, 119.
2. Ibid., chapter 13, 89.
3. *The Holy Bible*, Job 41:31–34.
4. Melville, *Moby Dick*, 548.
5. Hobbes, chapter 21, 153. While Hobbes argues that a subject may not break his contract with the sovereign, he may be released from it if the sovereign power loses the power to protect him. It is the "intention" of those who enter into the contract that Sovereignty be "immortall; yet is it in its own nature, not only subject to violent death, by foreign war, but also through the ignorance, and passions of men, it hath in it, from the very institution, many seeds of a natural mortality, by Intestine Discord."
6. Ibid., chapter 13, 90.
7. Hegel, *Phenomenology of Spirit*, #246. All references are to the paragraph numbers of the English edition.
8. Ibid., #187.
9. Hobbes, chapter 46, 469–70.
10. Ibid., 170.
11. Ibid., 142.
12. Hegel, #446–#476.
13. See Slaughter, *Human Rights, Inc.*, 4–5.
14. Anthony Woodiwiss argues, for example, that, while "the existing human rights regime" may have contributed to the idea of a global moral community, it appears to have become an "obstacle to the further development of such a moral community." Woodiwiss, *Human Rights*, 135. Woodiwiss links the success or failure of initiatives

based on human rights to the degree to which they threaten property rights; see p. 109. See also Galtung, *Human Rights in Another Key*. Galtung emphasizes the way in which the concept of rights is embedded in specific cultural commitments regarding personal liberty and nature that privilege property rights and political rights over economic and social justice.

15. Derrida, "From Restricted to General Economy," 252–53.

16. In 1800 only three U.S. states, Kentucky, Vermont, and New Hampshire, had universal white male suffrage.

17. Irigaray, *Je, Tu, Nous*, 22. Like Foucault, Irigaray deploys a critical method to reveal the historical specificity of the concept of Man, as well as the identities, institutions, and principles associated with it. Irigaray, however, recognizes the necessity of thinking through sexual difference, and, in doing so, forever subverts philosophy's reduction of difference to the One. Paying attention to the invisible and silent narratives of women's experience, as Irigaray proposes, may provide, as she often hopes, new figures of agency more adequate to promote health and happiness, a "livable future."

1. STATE OF NATURE!

1. Hobbes, *Leviathan*, chapter 6, 37–38.

2. Ibid., chapter 3, 21.

3. Ibid., chapter 6, 44.

4. Ibid.

5. Hobbes, *The Elements of Law*, chapter 12.2; all references are to paragraph numbers.

6. Ibid., chapter 12.5–12.6.

7. See Hobbes, *Leviathan*, chapter 3, 21.

8. Hobbes, *The Elements of Law*, chapter 14.6–14.7.

9. Ibid., chapter 14, 6.71.

10. See Blackstone's statement (1765) of the same argument in Blackstone, *Commentaries on the Laws of England*, 122.

11. Hobbes, *The Elements of Law*, chapter 14.10.

12. Hobbes, *Leviathan*, chapter 14, 91.

13. Philbrick, *Mayflower*, 101–2. Philbrick relates how Squanto gave the European settlers a "crash course in Indian agriculture," as their own attempts at cultivation were unsuccessful.

14. This absolute right informs the "Stand Your Ground" law in the U.S. state of Florida. The law authorizes the use of force whenever a man feels threatened.

15. See also chapter 6, 44–45. Here Hobbes identifies a voluntary action as beginning in appetite or fear. The difference between involuntary and voluntary actions as opposed to involuntary or voluntary wills hinges on the difference between man as speaking subject and man as a natural body. As a "necessity of nature," Man like any other natural body may be "pushed" or may "falleth." In voluntary actions, man acts upon appetite and fear. The voluntary will commits voluntary actions, but not every

voluntary action reflects a voluntary will. Hobbes' critique of opinion implies a certain rarity.

16. Hobbes, *The Elements of Law*, chapter 12, 6.

17. Hobbes, *Leviathan*, chapter 11, 76.

18. Hobbes, *The Elements of Law*, chapter 12, 7.

19. Hobbes, *Leviathan*, chapter 18, 120–21.

20. Hobbes, *The Elements of Law*, chapter 19.8.

21. The frontispiece makes clear Hobbes' insistence on the subordination of ecclesiastical power to sovereign power. See also his "Letter of January, 1650 to Robert Payne."

22. Hobbes, *Leviathan*, chapter 18, 125.

23. Woodiwiss, *Human Rights*, 9. See also page 31 on the primacy of the right to property.

24. Hobbes, *Leviathan*, chapter 6, 41; see also *The Elements of Law*, chapter 22.4.

25. Hobbes, *Leviathan*, chapter 4, 24.

26. A son remains dependent only until his reasoning capacity has developed sufficiently to ensure his self-reliance.

27. Hobbes, *Leviathan*, chapter 3, 21.

28. Ibid., chapter 5, 34.

29. Ibid., chapter 6, 42; see also chapter 3, 21.

30. See Joseph Slaughter's discussion of the "inconsistent" and "overdetermined" figure of the person in international law. Slaughter, *Human Rights, Inc.*, 19; see also 38–39. Slaughter exposes the way in which narrative is employed to legitimate social inequity.

31. Hobbes, *Leviathan*, chapter 4, 26.

32. Ibid., chapter 10, 65.

33. Ibid., chapter 5, 34.

34. Evans, *The Politics of Human Rights*, 53–54. Evans analyzes the way in which concerns about social justice are regularly trumped by market considerations. He demonstrates the complicity of human rights discourse in "lending legitimacy to the practices of global economic actors" that result in social, economic, and environmental injustice. Evans shows how "power is exercised through the discourse of human rights." If human rights discourse promises liberation, it also "offers an instrument for domination."

35. O'Neill, "Rights, Obligations, and World Hunger," 151.

36. This analysis of abstraction and its relation to the disposition of populations responds to Irigaray's proclamation of the "work" that is "needed" in "thought and ethics": "We need to reinterpret everything . . . beginning with the way in which the subject has always been written in the masculine form, as man, even when it claimed to be universal or neutral." Irigaray, *Ethics of Sexual Difference*, 6.

37. Hobbes, *Leviathan*, chapter 26, 213.

38. Hobbes, *Human Nature*, 4, 4.

39. *Leviathan*, chapter 5, 35. See also *The Elements of Law*, chapter 15.1.

40. *Leviathan*, chapter 5, 36.

41. Ibid., chapter 5, 36–37.

42. Jean-Jacques Rousseau, "Fifth Walk," in *Reveries of a Solitary Walker*, 85.

43. Rousseau, *Discourse on Inequality*, 2, 62.
44. Ibid., 2, 68; see also 61.
45. Rousseau, *The Social Contract*, 60.
46. Ibid., book 1, chapter 9, 67.
47. Ibid., book 2, chapter 4, 77.
48. Ibid., book 1, chapter 4, 61.
49. See Woodiwiss, *Human Rights*, 7.
50. Ibid.
51. Ibid., 136.
52. Rousseau, *The Social Contract*, book 1, chapter 9, 68. In *Emile* Rousseau is more cynical: "Those specious names, justice and order, will always serve as instruments of violence and as arms of iniquity." The very laws and institutions that are meant to sustain equality "serve to destroy it."
53. Rousseau, *The Social Contract*, 68.
54. Ibid., book 2, chapter 11, 96.
55. Ibid.
56. Macklin, "Reproductive Tourism in India."
57. In *Discourse on Inequality* Rousseau distinguishes three conditions: man's solitary, happy life in the state of nature; the brutish and violent competition with other men to which he is subject prior to the institution of the law of property; and his unhappy life under corrupt political institutions that convert "clever usurpation into an irrevocable right." Rousseau, *Discourse on Inequality*, 69. The "march of inequality" includes three stages: the establishment of law and the right of property, the institution of the magistrature or the bureaucracy for administering the law, and the transformation of legitimate into arbitrary power (ibid., 78). Man suffers prior to the contract from the threat of violence and after the contract from the inevitability of corruption. Political institutions are both necessary and dangerous. The first step toward inequality for Rousseau, as for Hobbes, is Man's propensity to compete for glory and prestige as much as for wealth (ibid., 61–62).
58. Rousseau, *The Social Contract*, book 2, chapter 4, 74.
59. Ibid., book 3, chapter 10, 135.
60. Ibid., 131.
61. Ibid., book 2, chapter 5, 78.
62. Rousseau, *Emile*, 52.
63. Ibid., 435.
64. Ibid., 52. See also Rousseau, *Discourse on Inequality*, 49, where a "savage" is said to be incapable of romantic love, because he is insensitive to "abstract ideas" of beauty and merit.
65. Rousseau, *Emile*, 53.
66. "By marriage, the husband and wife are one person in law: that is, the very being or legal existence of the woman is suspended during the marriage, or at least is incorporated and consolidated into that of the husband: under whose wing, protection, and *cover*,

she performs everything." From Blackstone, *Commentaries on the Laws of England*, 1.15, 430.

67. Wollstonecraft, *A Vindication of the Rights of Woman*.

68. The idea that the female sex provides an access to the universal that cannot be reduced to Man's runs throughout the philosophy of Luce Irigaray. Hillary Clinton gave the phrase contemporary force with her declaration that "women's rights are human rights" at the UN Conference on Women in Beijing in 1995.

69. Rousseau, *Emile*, book 5, 360.

70. Hegel, *Elements of the Philosophy of Right*, #203. References are to paragraph numbers.

71. Ibid., #166, *n2*.

72. "Takeout Foods, Restaurant Meals Tied to Obesity Trend."

73. Breen and Cook, "The Persistence of the Gendered Division of Labor."

74. Hersch, "Opting Out Among Women with Elite Education." See also Steiner, *Mommy Wars* and Lerner, *The War on Moms*.

2. CAPITALIZED BODIES

1. Rousseau, *Emile*, 370. *Frolic:* from D *vroolijk*, fr. MD *vrolijc*, fr. *Vro* happy; akin to OHG *frō* happy; 1538 full of fun, merry. All dictionary references are to *Merriam-Webster's Collegiate Dictionary*, 11th ed. (Springfield, MA: Merriam-Webster, 2014).

2. In his early texts, particularly *Madness and Civilization*, Foucault tends to equate power with repression. By the time of *Discipline and Punish*, he has come to understand that repression is not coextensive with power but only a type. Indeed, Foucault focuses increasingly on the productivity of power. It produces specific identities, forms of knowledge, and modes of social life. See "Foucault's Concept of Power: From Repression to Power/Knowledge," in Rawlinson, "Foucault's Strategy."

3. See Foucault, *Abnormal*, 244.

4. See Foucault, *Security, Territory, Population*, 70–71, 324–25.

5. Most bodies are commodified insofar as most humans live by selling their labor, thus becoming a unit cost in the apparatus of production and a commodity on the market like any other. Bodies are colonized when they are defined as the "other" within their home space, as the blacks of South Africa were displaced from the position of citizenship in their own country. A body is capitalized when the body itself becomes a profit center.

6. Though the concept of biopower is extracted from Foucault's texts, it is inflected differently here by being read in light of Luce Irigaray's analysis of the irreducibility of sexual difference.

7. Foucault, *The Birth of the Clinic*; *The Order of Things*; *Discipline and Punish*. Each text explores, in a specific realm of experience, the emergence at the end of the eighteenth century of new sciences and technologies for the management of bodies to maximize security and wealth. These infrastructures prefigure the management of populations under biopower.

8. Foucault, *Society Must Be Defended*, 240.

9. Sovereign power is always already marked male.
10. Foucault, *Society Must Be Defended*, 240.
11. See his discussion of the continuity of sovereign power and biopower, ibid., 242.
12. Oddly, Foucault rarely thematizes sexual difference, except in his critique of hetero-normativity. His perspective is invariably male: women appear as possible objects of male desire or as necessary complements in the prescriptions of masculinity. In his discussion of the importance of "the choice of love" in the Hellenistic and Roman "art of self-government," Foucault analyses the position of the masculine subject between a "love for women" and a "love for boys," but he never problematizes women's lack of subjectivity, that she is chosen, or not, but may never choose. Michel Foucault, "Subjectivity and Truth," 92. See also "The Social Triumph of the Sexual Will," 159: "We often say that the single person suffers from solitude because he is suspected of being an unsuccessful or rejected husband." In his account of the importance of virginity in self-government, Foucault does not distinguish between men's interest in their own virginity as an element of self-development and their interest in the virginity of women, about which he says relatively little. A man might take up celibacy to achieve detachment from life or to "recover the immortality of which one has been deprived" (Gregory of Nyssa). A man cares about the virginity of a woman out of a concern for his property. It ensures that the children who will inherit are *proper to him, his own*: thus, the prevalence throughout history of "tests" of virginity. Men's interest in the virginity of women is always motivated by a concern with the right to property, the ownership of children, and the security of inheritance. Foucault does note that, under Hellenistic and Roman theories of self-government, chaste women were respected as "virile" and credited with the same kind of self-regulation valorized in men. It is Christianity that grafts a logic of purity onto the idea of self-government, so that virginity as a "model of female integrity" becomes "much more important." In the matter of female virginity, the value of "physical integrity" displaces the virtue of self-regulation. She must be an unspoiled property to be of value. Her sexual integrity belongs to a man, not to herself. Foucault, "On the Genealogy of Ethics," 274.
13. Foucault, *Society Must Be Defended*, 247.
14. Foucault, *The Birth of the Clinic*, 196–97.
15. Adrien Proust's strategy of the *cordon sanitaire* exemplifies the importance of spatial distribution to health, to medicine, and to biopower. During a cholera epidemic in the 1890s, Dr. Proust, the father of Marcel, conceived and implemented the idea of spatially segregating the well and the ill with a policed barrier. Not surprisingly, these boundaries fell along social and economic lines. The idea was quickly appropriated by political discourse. In 1919 Clemenceau suggested that the chain of states separating Europe and Russia should serve as a *cordon sanitaire* between the two. Since then, the concept of "buffer states" has become common in political discourse.
16. Foucault, *Society Must Be Defended*, 243.
17. Ibid.

18. Cf. Agamben, *Homo Sacer*, 5. Foucault analyses how "the modern Western state has integrated techniques of subjective individualization with procedures of objective totalization . . . a 'double bind' created by individualization and the simultaneous totalization of structures of modern power."

19. Foucault, *Security, Territory, Population*, 108.

20. Foucault, *The Birth of Biopolitics*, 220–28. Foucault distinguishes between the abstract analysis of labor in terms of wage or the "factor of time" in classical economics and the idea of human lives as sites of investments for the production of future income streams in neoliberalism. If the theory of human capital is only articulated in the work of post–World War II economists, the practice of treating human lives as capital is at least as old as modernity. See, for example, Henry James' study of the investments made in a young girl by an ambitious mother in order to ensure her economic success in the marriage market: "I have raised money on that girl's face." James, *Roderick Random*, 295–96, 404–5.

21. Foucault, *Ethics*, 69.

22. Foucault, *Security, Territory, Population*, 69. See also 108.

23. Ibid., 69.

24. Ibid., 70.

25. Foucault, *Abnormal*, 240.

26. Barker-Benfield, *Horrors of the Half-Known Life*, 166, 176–81. See also Engelhardt, "The Disease of Masturbation."

27. Foucault, *Abnormal*, 241.

28. Ibid. On this "universal causality," Foucault cites the essay by Fournier and Bégin on "Masturbation" in the *Dictionnaire des sciences médicales* published in Paris in 1819.

29. Quoted in Duffy, "Masturbation and Clitoridectomy," 246.

30. Freud, *Civilization and Its Discontents*, 21:97.

31. Freud, Lecture XXI, *Introductory Lectures on Psychoanalysis*, 16:329.

32. See Rawlinson, "Psychoanalytic Discourse and the Feminine Voice."

33. Foucault, *Abnormal*, 250.

34. Ibid., 255.

35. Ibid., 248. In another sign of his blindness to sexual difference and female subjectivity, Foucault writes "parents'" here, not "mothers.'" The treatise to which he refers, however, Rozier's *Des habitudes secretes ou des maladies produites par l'onanisme chez les femmes*, published in Paris in 1830, specifically names the mother. It is she who "puts them [her children] in her flesh."

36. Ibid., 257–58.

37. As Foucault notes, the campaign against masturbation and the regulation of the family focused not only on the surveillance of children but also on the surveillance of household labor. He quotes Deslandes' 1832 treatise *De l'onanisme*: "We are especially suspicious of female domestics; since we confide young children to their care, they often seek in them compensation for their forced celibacy." Foucault, *Abnormal*, 244.

The hierarchies of property and social inequity remain intertwined with the ideologies and technologies of sexuality and gender.

38. Ibid., 245.

39. Ibid., 247.

40. "Salzman's fight against masturbation was conducted as a battle for the nation." Stengers and van Neck, *Masturbation*, 89. Christian Gotthilf Salzmann was a German theologian and reformer who subscribed to Philanthropinism, an educational program based on Rousseau's philosophy. Salzman modeled his school on the family. Like many of his peers, he frequently sounded the alarm about the dangers of onanism. Toilets were of particular concern and required extensive surveillance and regulation, as he considered them "tombs of innocence."

41. Stengers and van Neck, *Masturbation*, 85.

42. Ibid., 86.

43. Foucualt, *Abnormal*, 250.

44. Ibid., 144.

45. Ibid., 253.

46. Ehrenreich and English, *Complaints and Disorders*, 34.

47. See Moscucci, *The Science of Woman*, 30–32. See also Groneman, "The Historical Construction of Female Sexuality," 339. Nymphomania was associated with not only a variety of sexual and "nervous complaints" but also with malaria or pulmonary disease, as well as, at least by one doctor, with having blonde hair. Groneman argues that these nineteenth-century theories ascribing a ubiquitous causality to the sexual functions marked a radical departure in medicine from the Aristotelian theory of woman as a malformed man. This "one-sex model" gives way to theories that maintain man as the generically human, while casting women as fundamentally different beings. While sexuality may exert a ubiquitous influence over him, a man still possesses the full range of human capacities and is determined by multiple causalities, including his own agency. Multiple sciences will be necessary to understand man, while gynecology covers a woman's whole being.

48. Barker-Benfield, *Horrors of the Half-Known Life*, 83.

49. Quoted in Ehrenreich and English, *Complaints and Disorders*, 28.

50. For an account of the extent to which the figure of the invalid has mediated women's identity in the United States, see Herndl, *Invalid Women*.

51. Gilman, *The Yellow Wallpaper*.

52. Moscucci, *The Science of Woman*, 104, 107–8.

53. Foucault, *The History of Sexuality*, 1:141.

54. Ibid.

55. Ibid.

56. Weiss-Wolf, "My Daughter Was Dress-Coded for Wearing Shorts." See also "Dress Code Debate Heats Up Around the Country." In this report the discussants quickly dismiss any objections to the codes. See also Sadikman, "A Dress Code of Her Own."

57. Hochman, "Protest at Morris Knolls HS."

58. See, however, research indicating that markets misunderstand Norwegian girls, who do not want to look "sexy," but *kul*. As the sexualized look is purveyed for girls as young as three, it is likely that the girls' sexualized styles reflect the power of the market, rather than a personal style. Rysst, "'I Am Only Ten Years Old.'"

59. Keltner, "The Top 12 Fall Fashion Trends 2009."

60. Durisin, "12 Sexed-up Brands that Market to Teens." See also Cruz, "Adidas Targets Teenage Girls."

61. Irigaray, *Je, Tu, Nous*, 76; see also her *Thinking the Difference*, 15, 71–72.

62. Chandler, "Revealing Look at Preteen Chic." See also Moisse, "10-Year-Old Model's Grown-up Look."

63. Baudrillard, *The Consumer Society*, 89. See also Baudrillard's definition of consumption as "an active, collective behavior . . . something enforced, a morality, an institution . . . a whole system of values, with all that expression implies in terms of group integration and social control functions" (81).

64. "Women's Clothing Stores in the U.S."

65. http://s79.photobucket.com/user/motownnat/media/eva-mendes-sexy-lingerie -Calvin-Kle.jpg.html.

66. Odell, "Spring 2009's Most Dangerous Shoes."

67. Cunningham, "On the Street."

68. Cosmetic foot surgery is a growing market in the United States. Castillo, "Women Undergoing Foot Surgery." See also Saltzberg and Chrisler, "Beauty Is the Beast."

69. "Several Models Fall During Hervé Léger Show."

70. There appears to be very little work, theoretical or practical, focusing on the rights of these models, but there is a plethora of websites devoted to making fun of them and taking pleasure in their humiliation. Even some mainstream news media have indulged in cruel and demeaning reporting, positioning these incidents as occasions for derisive laughter rather than for an analysis of labor injustice. See, for example, "News reader cannot stop laughing at model falling over!" (YouTube).

71. See "Several Models Fall."

72. Borrelli-Persson, "Runway Review."

73. Campbell, "Models Reveal Why They Need a Union."

74. Lunt et al., "Medical Tourism," 14.

75. Singh, "Budget 2003–2004."

76. Apollo Hospitals Enterprise Ltd., http://www.apollohospitals.com.

77. Narayan, "Challenges of the National Rural Health Mission."

78. National Guidelines for Accreditation, Supervision, and Regulation of ART Clinics in India, http://ww.icmr.nic.in/art/Chapter_3.pdf; Gupta, "Reproductive Biocrossings," 33.

79. Ballantyne, "Exploitation in Cross-Border Reproductive Care," 94.

80. Quoted in Warner, "Outsourced Wombs."

81. See Jaggar, "Global Responsibility and Western Feminism." Jaggar criticizes cultural critique when it is unhinged from any analysis of the institutions and powers of global

capital. She cites "the way in which women in the global South suffer disproportionately from the interlocking problems of sexualization, militarism, and environmental destruction," which reflect the interests of "neoliberal globalization."

82. Like Jaggar, Foucault identifies the effects of global capital with American neoliberalism, which "extends the rationality of the market, the schemes of analysis it proposes, and the decisionmaking criteria it suggests to areas that are not exclusively or not primarily economic. For example, the family and birth policy, or delinquency and penal policy." Foucault, *The Birth of Biopolitics*, 78.

83. Carolyn Mcleod has argued that an infrastructure of pressures and expectations around biological reproduction makes Anglo-European women vulnerable to market forces. She questions the morality of dedicating resources to surrogacy, while many children exist who lack parents. Mcleod argues that developing transnational adoption programs is a more morally defensible policy response to infertility than surrogacy. On the "right to reproduce," see Botterell and Mcleod, "Can a Right to Reproduce Justify the Status Quo in Parental Licensing?"

84. Macklin, "Is There Anything Wrong with Surrogate Motherhood?"

85. Macklin, "Reproductive Tourism in India." Angela Ballantyne also argues against the claim of exploitation on the grounds that, while the relation between client and surrogate is mutually advantageous, there are no clear criteria for determining what would count as a fair distribution of benefits and hence no way of determining whether the surrogate is being exploited. This abstract, definitional analysis pays no attention to the complicity of state power and capital in the recruiting and marketing of the surrogates. See Ballantyne, "Exploitation in Cross-Border Reproductive Care."

86. Gestational surrogacy requires an extensive regimen of hormone treatments to prepare the surrogate to receive the fertilized embryo. Through the nine months of pregnancy, she is subject to dramatic alterations that affect every element of her embodiment, including her mobility. Depending on the nature of the birth, she requires some period of recovery. Throughout she is subject to the possibility of more or less serious complications, without any long-term insurance. If the industry is not taking her life, it is certainly "making [her] live" to the advantage of global capital. Unlike the hard labor to which Macklin compares it, this labor uniquely involves the laborer's whole body, permits no break for at least a year, and offers no opportunity of changing one's mind.

87. Given the potential for exploitation, some feminist bioethicists have argued against transnational surrogacy and in favor of "national self-sufficiency," but as long as there is a "market" in "gestational services," the same problems of inequity and exploitation will reappear in the national context. See Kane and Martin, "National Self-Sufficiency in Reproductive Resources."

88. Foucault, "The Social Triumph of the Sexual Will," 158.

89. Surrogacy is labor, but a unique form, so that a critique of commodification is not adequate to address it. See also Crozier, Johnson, and Hajzler, "At the Intersections of Emotional and Biological Labor." Crozier and her colleagues treat surrogacy as labor

and suggest that the market may be the best context in which to make visible the value of the emotional and biological labor of reproduction. Though they do not fully appreciate the uniqueness of generative labor, they propose an intervention that recognizes and addresses the transnational inequities underlying transnational surrogacy.

90. Irigaray, "Human Nature is Two," 39.

91. This does not imply that all mothers are good mothers, but most mothers are, in Winnicott's famous formulation, "good enough"; most mothers want to see their children become free agents. See Winnicott, *Playing and Reality*, 10–11, 81.

92. Foucault, "What Is Enlightenment?" 319, 316.

93. Foucault, "The Masked Philosopher," 325.

94. Cf. Elizabeth Grosz's account of the reconceptualization of life in Darwin's thought: "life is now construed, perhaps for the first time, as fundamental becoming, becoming without the definitive features of (Aristotelian) being, without a given (Platonic) form. . . . Tied to neither the natural nor the social spheres alone, the concept of life now serves as a bridge, a point of connection and transition between the biological and the cultural, the ways in which matter opens itself up to social transformation, and the ways in which social change works with and through biologically open, individual and collective, bodies." Grosz, *Time Travels*, 37.

95. Foucault, "The Masked Philosopher," 323.

96. Ibid.

97. Ibid.

98. Foucault, "What Is Enlightenment?" 315–16.

99. See Foucault on the "end of man" in *The Order of Things*, 386–87.

100. Foucault, "What Is Enlightenment?" 311.

101. Heidegger, *Being and Time*; Sartre, *Being and Nothingness*.

102. See, e.g., Butler, *Gender Trouble*, especially section 4 of part 3 and the conclusion.

103. Foucault, *The Birth of the Clinic*, 198.

104. Ibid., 197.

105. See Derrida's discussion of the constitution of the ideality of language by "my-death." Derrida, *Speech and Phenomena*, 54. "The appearing of the I to itself in the *I am* is thus originally a relation with its own possible disappearance. Therefore, *I am* originally means *I am mortal. I am immortal* is an impossible proposition."

II: REFIGURING ETHICS

1. Jane Austen's novels provide a study of the marriage market, while those of Charles Dickens, later in the nineteenth century, often analyze the institution of the "work house," by which the poor were to be made productive.

2. Hobbes, *Leviathan*, chapter 10, 63.

3. Despite Foucault's contrast between German ordoliberalism and American neoliberalism on this point, capitalism, in all its forms, involves the management of life to produce wealth and security. This is certainly true in Germany, where state policy

carefully manages health and reproduction to promote productivity and wealth. Cf. Foucault, *The Birth of Biopolitics*, 219.

4. See Folbre, *Valuing Children*.

3. ANTIGONE AND ISMENE

1. Derrida, "Différance," 19; see also his "From Restricted to General Economy," 251–52. "To laugh at philosophy (at Hegelianism)."

2. Hegel, *Phenomenology of Spirit*, #429–76.

3. Benhabib, "Multiculturalism and Gendered Citizenship," 97. Benhabib likens her to the three young Muslim women of North African origin and French citizenship who wore head scarves to school in spite of state ordinances against the display of private religious symbols in public space: "Like Antigone . . . these young girls used the symbols of the private realm to challenge the ordinances of the public sphere." Like Uighur women in China, these girls used the veil to protest the repression of their cultures. These examples make clear the complexity of the politics of women's dress. The same garment can be a sign of subjection or of agency. The issue for ethics and politics is not the garment but with whom decisions about a woman's dress reside: with her? In what culture of possibilities does a woman dress?

4. These claims are particularly important to Judith Butler's reading of Antigone. See Butler, *Antigone's Claim*, 82.

5. Benhabib, "On Hegel, Women, and Irony," 255.

6. Butler, *Antigone's Claim*, 61.

7. At l. 347 in *Oedipus at Colonus*, Oedipus insults his sons by calling them womanish, while acknowledging that Ismene and Antigone have exhibited a filial devotion. This passage might seem to support readings that focus on gender transgression; however, the aim of Oedipus' insult is to deride his sons for their lack of loyalty to him. They have sided with the power of the state over their filial bond. Oedipus is the kind of man given to name-calling, and here he employs a tired line of the schoolyard bully, calling his sons "girls." In fact, all the siblings, except Ismene, who exhibits an unusual agency in *Oedipus at Colonus*, adhere strictly to their gender-defined duties, Antigone caring for the body, and the men going to war over property, power, and pride. See note 17, this chapter.

8. Irigaray, *Speculum of the Other Woman*, 217.

9. Indeed, with one exception, the only positive interpretation of Ismene I was able to find I discovered on www.sparknotes.com: "Ismene—Blonde, full-figured, and radiantly beautiful, the laughing, talkative Ismene is the good girl of the family. She is reasonable and understands her place, bowing to Creon's edict and attempting to dissuade Antigone from her act of rebellion. Antigone—The play's tragic heroine. Antigone is opposed to her radiant sister Ismene. Unlike her beautiful and docile sister, Antigone is scrawny, sallow, withdrawn, and recalcitrant brat." A caution to students not to trust summaries.

10. Mills, "Hegel's *Antigone*," 72.

11. Ibid.

12. Ibid., 71–72. Among commentators, only Bonnie Honig veers from this well-trodden path of valorizing one sister at the expense of the other. Honig's acute reading focuses on the fact that there are *two* burials in *Antigone*. She not only offers a positive account of Ismene's character and agency but also casts Antigone as acting on behalf of her sister. There is an element of mystery in Honig's hefty account that I do not want to spoil. Let me say only that, if her rendering of the burials were correct, there would be no reason for Antigone, Ismene, and Haemon not to conspire to prevent Antigone's death. Indeed, Haemon and Ismene are successful in moving Creon to relent, but Antigone *has already embraced death*. See Honig, "Ismene's Forced Choice," 29; see also her *Antigone Interrupted*, chapter 6.

13. Though Hegel's concept of life focuses on human life or history, it incorporates Earth and all that is subject to a logic of generation. Life "has its death within itself," as its own growth and development is also always a passing away. Hegel distinguishes Life as a form from both the flux of life, or becoming, and the specific identity of the living being. The form of *human* life is the "I," agency, or the "category of action." The flux of human life, its process, or form of becoming, is history. And the specific identity of the living human being consists in understanding experience as action, that is, in assuming the narrative position, but only in order to relinquish it to the one who comes after. In Hegel's account the individual must come to accept himself as "only an instance." What compensates for this loss of life, in his analysis, is nothing beyond experience. Neither an "alien power" nor any other mysterious machinery of transubstantiation can be invoked by the philosopher to qualify the evidence of the putrefying corpse, for a transubstantiation *has indeed taken place*. The other, this one with whom I shared breath, food and drink, the warmth of the sun, has become an impossible presence. Hegel finds compensation in a *terrestrial faith*, in his belief in Earth as the "immortal individual," of which the single human being can be only a moment and which will live on after his death. Unfortunately, in our time, the mortality of Earth is all too palpable.

14. Philosophy in the West, including political philosophy, is built upon the foundation of a mythological violence: from the Greeks to Hobbes and Hegel to Freud and Lévi-Strauss, the brothers kill the father in order to redistribute his wealth, his property, and his women. Fraternity is installed as the controlling political structure to contain the violence and protect the privileges of property. Henceforth, patriarchy is set within it. The father's authority over the family depends on the recognition of it by other male heads-of-household. The lateral relations of fraternity sustain the vertical or hierarchical relations of patriarchy. Thus feminism misses its target when it identifies patriarchy as the sustaining structure of subjection.

15. Call him the *fraternal*, as opposed to the primal, father.

16. Irigaray, *Speculum of the Other Woman*, 225. See also her *This Sex Which Is Not One*. "Without the exploitation of the body-matter of women, what would become of the

symbolic process that governs society? What modifications would this process, this society, undergo, if women were to become 'speaking subjects' as well? . . . An other, that would be woman, still seems, in its terms, unimaginable" (ibid., 85).

17. Sophocles, *Oedipus at Colonus* (trans. Storr), l. 1368. Here Oedipus refers to *both* sisters as "men." This passage too might seem to support Butler's thesis of gender transgression—*but for both sisters*. In fact, it only reflects Oedipus' intention to sneer at his son, his "murderer," by impugning his manhood, as he did also at the beginning of the play. This is no less a schoolyard taunt than that. It reflects not only Oedipus' anger at the son who has put power above filial duty but also his identification of the virtue of faithfulness with manliness. When a woman is faithful, it is exceptional, manlike. See also note 7, this chapter.

18. Hobbes, *Leviathan*, chapter 13, 88–89.

19. Srebrenica, Bosnia, July 1995.

20. Boko Haram, Nigeria, April 2014.

21. Mukhtar Mai, Meerwala, Pakistan 2002.

22. Judging him a traitor, Creon decrees that Polyneices' body be left "unburied, to be meat for dogs and carrion crows" (*Antigone* l. 203). Later, Thebes is again subject to a miasma when its altars are fouled by the excretions and regurgitations of the animals that have eaten Polyneices' flesh (*Antigone* ll. 1017–18).

23. Sophocles, *Antigone* (trans. Storr), ll. 450–70.

24. See Pinkard, *Hegel's Phenomenology*, 140–41. "By carrying out the proper burial rites, the family members protect the standing of the deceased in the public community (the *Gemeinwesen*), for they signal by this that his *self*-identity remains important, not just his natural existence." The burial rite and other customs transform the contingency of "natural" or biological relations into "ethical" relationships in which certain things *must be done*. The "absolute duty" of family members figures the emergence of ethical life in and through natural life.

25. Hegel's *Phenomenology of Spirit* argues for the moral imperative that the individual ought to identify himself with the long-term interests of the species, even if that requires sacrificing what seem to be his short-term interests. "At a time when the universality of Spirit has gathered such strength . . . when too that universal aspect claims and holds on to the whole range of the wealth it has developed, the share in the total work of Spirit which falls to the individual can only be very small. . . . He must make of himself and achieve what he can; but less must be demanded of him, just as he in turn can expect less of himself, and may demand less for himself" (preface, #72, ibid.).

26. Irigaray, "The Eternal Irony of the Community," 217.

27. Ibid.

28. *Oedipus at Colonus*, ll.1408, 1435.

29. Transcendence is a nontheological concept of the experience of oneself as participating in a community of collaborative practices and institutions that are effective in sustaining and promoting life. A scientist transcends himself by participating in specific and material ways in the scientific community, just as a legislator transcends

herself by exercising a vote that is not merely her own but one authorized by her constituency.

30. Hegel, *Elements of the Philosophy of Right*, #166, note 2.

31. Women live in the "atmosphere of representational thought." Ibid.

32. See Rawlinson, "Beyond Virtue and the Law."

33. Hegel, *Phenomenology of Spirit*, #434.

34. Ibid., #431.

35. Ibid., #429.

36. Ibid., #437.

37. Sophocles, *Antigone* (trans. Storr), l. 1028. Of course, Creon's stupid stubbornness is typical of the oedipal family. Both Oedipus, in the first play, and Polyneices, in the second, obstinately refuse wise counsel to disastrous results. (*Antigone* was Sophocles first play, and *Oedipus at Colonus* his last. I refer to the plays in their order of presentation as determined by the narrative.)

The argument between Creon and Haemon is another passage that might seem to support a reading of the play around the theme of gender transgression, but Creon's stupid suggestion that forgiving Antigone would somehow threaten his authority is just that, and treated as such by Haemon. Haemon belittles his father's concern that "she would appear the man and I the woman" as evidence of Creon's lack of "manhood," rudely addressing his father as "boy." It is not that Antigone "is male" or even masculine, but that Creon denies her distinctively female agency and proves himself childish, a petulant "boy," in doing so. See also notes 7 and 17, this chapter.

38. Hegel, *Phenomenology of Spirit*, #468.

39. It is worth remembering that Polyneices has a legitimate grievance against his brother Eteocles, even as he displays the typical oedipal hardness of head and heart in responding to it. The twin brothers, after rescinding their original decision to yield the rule of Thebes to Creon, agree to share its rule on a rotating basis and to determine which brother will rule first on the basis of a coin toss. Eteocles, the younger brother, wins and serves his term, but when it comes time to relinquish the throne to Polyneices he refuses. Polyneices, having married the princess of Argos, assembles a force to assail Thebes. Both brothers exhibit the same choleric temper, rash judgment, lack of mercy, and tendency to blame others that define their father. While one might not be able to accept at face value Oedipus' indignation over Polyneices' lack of filial devotion, given his own paternal failings, it is nonetheless clear that Polyneices holds others as units in a calculus of advantage. He will use his father to advance his political ambitions, just as he will use his sister to cover his mortal vulnerabilities. In both cases his nearest human being is a unit in a calculus of power. Eteocles and Creon exhibit the same logic.

40. Is this hardness not evident in the uncharitable readings of Ismene?

41. In Hegel's account it is at once necessary to dethrone the family and to provide for its autonomous sphere of action. Only then will the antagonism and confusion of state and family be resolved. Of course, this depends on organizing human life by the logic

of man and woman, the normative roles of gender prescribed by fraternity and based in mythic violence and the right to property.

42. Irigaray, *Speculum of the Other Woman*, 224.

43. It is not too soon to notice that even a successful disruption of Hegel's normative system of gender does not dispense with the need for material infrastructures to support both work *and* family, both public and private forms of solidarity. How this is to be accomplished without relying on the difference of gender, as Hegel does, remains a question most often answered by new difficulties like latchkey children or a reliance on undocumented labor. In both scholarship and public policy, sexual difference remains a contested site not only because of the contestation of specific gender norms but most intractably because of the lack of material infrastructures adequate to sustain the complexity of human generativity. The painful pertinence today of the problem of integrating work and family only confirms the truth of this Hegelian analysis.

44. Ibid., 219.

45. Ibid., 217–18. Psychoanalytic prejudices lead many commentators astray, but no one veers farther from the plays than Irigaray in her caricature of Ismene and sanctification of Antigone.

46. Sophocles, *Oedipus at Colonus*, l. 1108.

47. Sophocles, *Oedipus at Colonus*, ll. 1700ff., particularly the last line, "her love and mine." The chorus confirms the respect due these "best of daughters" and venerates both sisters and their solidarity, addressing them as a "worthy pair."

48. Sophocles, *Oedipus at Colonus*, l. 354.

49. Ibid., l. 313.

Aetna, daughter of Gaia by her son Uranus, arbitrated between Demeter and Haephestus in a dispute over Sicily. She contains both the monstrous Typhon or Enceladus and the place where Zeus' thunderbolts are made. Aetna may be the place of Persephone's rape. Aetna is sometimes said to be the daughter of Poseidon and hence associated with horses, as well as the coupling of Poseidon and Demeter in the form of horses after the rape of Persephone. She is the mother of the Palikoi, who provide sanctuary for runaway slaves.

50. I am indebted to my colleague Sara Lipton in the Department of History at Stony Brook University for making me attentive to the hat.

51. Smith, *A Dictionary of Greek and Roman Antiquities*, 2:428.

52. Winckelmann, *The History of Ancient Art*, 2:23.

53. Hobbes, *Leviathan*, 88. The whole wretched history begins with a young man and an old man fighting over precedence at a bridge. The story is very familiar, but it is a strange, mad scene, a mad drama in a landscape of horror, where men rape and kill in the name of honor.

54. Again, Honig's analysis challenges this claim, but it is not clear that Antigone's death was in any sense necessary or unavoidable, even if we ascribe to her a different intention, one that would serve life, rather than only the burial of Polyneices.

55. If Antigone means to make a political intervention, as feminist authors regularly suggest, then what is her plan? To what end does she act? Her refusal to submit to Creon's

decree does not serve the future nor does it generate any political solidarity that might serve her community. In what sense is her suicide "a form of defiance against patriarchal domination" (Mills, "Hegel's Antigone," 74) when its only result is the abandonment of the sister and the future?

56. In *Oedipus at Colonus* she interprets for Oedipus both the oracle's pronouncement and the intentions of his Theban relatives. See ll. 363–421.

57. Sophocles, *Antigone* (trans. Grene and Lattimore), l. 578. Once again, it is Ismene who has transgressed the norms of womanhood by running around. Remarkably, Irigaray does comment on this passage. She argues that the imprisonment of Ismene is evidence that she is just another woman to be shut up in the house, while Antigone's exceptionalism is evident in her willingness to kill herself so that "her brother, *her mother's desire*, may have eternal life." Irigaray ignores not only the threat to Creon posed by Ismene's effective agency, but also Antigone's willful exposure of her deed. Antigone clearly demonstrates that it is not so much Polyneices' eternal life as her own willfulness that is at stake here.

58. Ibid., l. 568.

59. Had Creon allowed the burial of both brothers or had he forgiven Antigone, there would not have been a third play. Creon is guilty of producing Antigone's disobedience with the bad decree that offends familial obligation to no purpose, especially as Polyneices had a legitimate claim against his brother as ruler of Thebes. It is Creon's stupid and stubborn adherence to his belief that a decree once uttered can never be rescinded, lest his manliness be compromised, that wreaks havoc. Of course, as Haemon argues, it is just this intransigence that renders him a boy rather than a man. Once more, Cadmean hardheadedness and hardheartedness cause disaster.

60. Sophocles, *Antigone*, l. 100.

61. Sophocles, *Antigone* (Lattimore), l. 548.

62. *Oedipus at Colonus*, ll. 1415–45.

63. Sophocles, *Antigone* (Lattimore), ll. 540–52.

64. Ibid., l. 567.

65. Ibid., l. 558.

66. Sabrina Hom's analysis of mourning in *Antigone* prompted me to notice the importance of this moment in which Ismene mourns Antigone's death while her sister is still alive. Hom, "Antigone Falters."

67. Sophocles, *Oedipus at Colonus*, ll. 592ff.

68. Ibid., ll. 566–67.

69. Sophocles, *Antigone* (Lattimore), l. 1291.

70. Prefigured here in the power of the lord over life and death is the power of the state to submit the individual to its judgment not only through juridical power over life and death but also through pervasive normative practices that shape and contain life.

71. The murder of the *primal* father (Laius) occurs outside time, both outside of history and outside of the plays.

72. Sophocles, *Oedipus at Colonus*, l. 1670.

73. Chandler, *The Simple Art of Murder*, 17.

74. While the terms *matricide*, *fratricide*, and *patricide* are familiar, the term *sororicide*, though it exists, is relatively unusual and does not appear in standard dictionaries, as if the sacrifice of the daughter or sister, on which not only Greek culture but also the rights of man depend, were invisible.

75. The marriage of a mature man to a young girl would have been commonplace, as it often is even today. Due to the laws of property and the frequency of death in childbirth, a girl of thirteen or fourteen might be married to a man in his forties or fifties who had already had one or more wives. His sons from previous marriages might be more nearly his wife's age, and no doubt their youth would attract her own. If we make Oedipus as young as possible, in order to make Jocasta no older than we must, we may estimate that Jocasta was fourteen when she married Laius, who was forty-five. Eighteen years later, he is sixty-three when killed by the youth Oedipus and Jocasta thirty-two. Many years pass before the *krisis* of the miasma. Laius' death is said to have occurred long ago. If we assume twenty years between the two periods, Jocasta is in her early fifties and Oedipus barely forty at the beginning of the plays. In *Oedipus Rex* his sons are grown men, his daughters girls. Another twenty years or so pass between the first and second plays. In *Oedipus at Colonus* the twins Polyneices and Eteocles must be at least in their late thirties or early forties, while Antigone and Ismene cannot be younger than their mid twenties in the second and third plays, long past the usual age of marriage. Life has been passing them by.

4. DEMETER AND PERSEPHONE

1. See Rawlinson, "The Right to Life." See also Woodiwiss, *Human Rights*, 7, 9, 31, 109, 135.

2. The underrepresentation of women in the counsels that determine the future is virtually ubiquitous. Globally, women have very little presence in the decision-making bodies of government, academia, and business. Women have been allowed to vote in Western countries for barely more than a century. Women account for just 5 percent of CEOs in Fortune 500 companies. There are three female CEOs in the FTSE 100. Although law and medical school classes in the United States had reached gender parity by 2003, in 2010 women still comprised only 13 percent of medical school deans, 20 percent of law school deans, and 23 percent of university presidents. Moreover, women tend to lead less prestigious institutions and to serve shorter terms than men. See White et al., "Gender-Related Differences." In 2013 women held 18.3 percent of seats in the U.S. House of Representatives and 20 percent of seats in the U.S. Senate, 23 percent of seats in the UK House of Commons, and 33 percent of seats in the European Parliament. In China women hold 21 percent of the seats in the National People's Congress. In China's State Council only 3 of 28 ministers or commissioners are women. In many countries in South Asia and the Middle East, women continue to live under tribal systems of gender subjection that result in significant disadvantages in education, nutrition, and health care. In "The Global Gender Gap Report 2012" of the World Economic Forum, only 15 of 135 countries score above .75 with 1.0

representing gender equity. These include eleven European countries, the Philippines, Nicaragua, New Zealand, and Lesotho.

Women's bodies and sexuality are regularly made subservient to capital and used to sell everything from soap to cars. See also Kilbourne, "Beauty . . ." In many developing countries, such as India, women's bodies have become profit centers in the state's effort to produce foreign capital. See Gupta, "Reproductive Biocrossings."

In tribal societies in South Asia and the Middle East, women's bodies literally become the battlegrounds in disputes among men. See, e.g., the case of Mukhtaran Bibi: on the orders of her all-male village council, her body was made the means of restoring honor to a family offended by the attentions of her twelve-year-old brother to one of its daughters. Various facts in the case are disputed, including whether or not she was gang-raped or rather forced to have sex with a male from the offended family. In either scenario, her body was made the site of the battle between the two families. See, e.g., http://www.bbc.co.uk/news/world-south-asia-13205439. But see also http://www.thenews.com.pk/Todays-News-9-44406-Mukhtaran-Mai-the-other-side-of-the-story.

In many Western societies, such as the United States, women are far more vulnerable to violence, particularly domestic violence, than are men. According to the U.S. Center for Disease Control and Prevention, one out of every four women in the United States has experienced domestic violence in her lifetime, while 85 percent of intimate partner violence in the United States is directed against women. See http://www.cdc.gov/violenceprevention/intimatepartnerviolence/datasources.html.

3. See Figure 4.1. Gaia is regularly depicted in this position. See also Attic red-figured *hydria*, attributed to the Oinanthe Painter, British Museum Vase E182. Later, she is represented prostrate at Uranus' feet: see, e.g., Aion Mosaic, Glyptothek Munich.

4. Hesiod, *Theogony*, 188.

5. Chronus curses his son with the fear that, like his father, Zeus too will be supplanted by his own son. Zeus, in turn, tries to block the generativity of Metis by eating her; however, the logic of patricide has been suspended, and the productive maternal force cannot be contained. Zeus cannot contain Metis' child, who like a hatching chick pecking at the eggshell, tap, tap, taps at Zeus' skull with the tip of her spear until she cracks it open and makes her exit/entrance.

6. *The Odyssey of Homer*, book 1, 282, book 2, 216.

7. Hobbes, *Leviathan*, 88. "Gain" includes any increase in wealth or power, not only the acquisition of property per se.

8. Hegel, *Phenomenology of Spirit*, 455.

9. *The Odyssey of Homer*, book 11, 474–76.

10. Ibid., 488–91.

11. See, e.g., Demeter of Knidos, ca. 350 BCE, London, British Museum, or the statue of Demeter discovered at Herculaneum, April 21, 1997, and now in the Museo Archeologico Nazionale di Napoli.

12. See Calasso, *The Marriage of Cadmus and Harmony*. Reading Calasso's text made me realize that I could retell these stories in my own way for my own ends, as authors have done for millennia. While everything I recount appears in some author, I have recon-

structed the stories to expose the lies and misrepresentations of Zeus and his authors and to reveal again the agency of the two mothers.

13. The field is said to be "thrice-plowed." This figure has at least three implications. First, Demeter herself embodies the generations of her mothers and is intrinsically three. Second, the drama of Demeter and Persephone will be resolved in the threesome of three generations: (grand)mother, the daughter who is also a mother, and the son. Finally, Dionysus is himself "thrice-born."

14. To farm: to raise another living being for the purpose of eating it or selling it to others who will eat it.

15. Ovid, *Metamorphosis*, book 9, ll. 420–23.

16. Kerényi, *Eleusis*, 147. The phrase "abyss of the seed" (*Abgrund des Kerns*) is from Goethe.

17. After Metaneira interrupted her at the fire, where she was burning away Demophoon's mortal flesh, Demeter threw him to the ground and left the house of Celeus. It is said that the child was never again happy, as he always missed the radiant presence of his nurse, the goddess.

18. She gives no evidence, but Irigaray claims that Aphrodite and Demeter represent "two eras of gynocratic rule." Both Aphrodite and Demeter, however, live under the fraternal order of the three brothers. Irigaray also suggests that, while Aphrodite represents "natural growth and love," Demeter represents "the mother within marriage." She contrasts the earth's "spontaneous" "fruitfulness" and "flowering" under Aphrodite, whom she links to "water, dampness," with the domestication of the earth under Demeter through agriculture and the cycle of seasons. In fact, the stories of Aphrodite suggest that she was a deceitful troublemaker who loved to sow discord and strife, while those of Demeter emphasize her readiness to enjoy life and nurture others. See Irigaray, *Sexes and Genealogies*, 129.

19. As in the ekstasis of the dithyramb, all this happens at once in myth: the mother has always already lost her child(hood), and the daughter/maiden has always already been violated.

20. See, e.g., the Dancers' Frieze from the Building of the Dancers' Frieze or Temnos at the Samothrace Temple Complex or Sanctuary of the Great Gods. The frieze is specifically associated with Persephone, just as the practices of the sanctuary itself privileged the veneration of Demeter.

21. Foley, *The Homeric Hymn to Demeter*, ll. 417–28.

22. Hesiod catalogues the Oceanides in *Theogony*. Hesiod, *Theogony*, ll. 346–70. It was Brown's comment in his introduction which made me pay attention to their "allegorically significant names."

23. *Respect*: from Latin *respectus*, the act of looking back.

24. Calasso's confusion here leads him to describe Hades as the "eye par excellence," but that title belongs indisputably to Zeus whose powers of surveillance are unequaled (Calasso, *The Marriage of Cadmus and Harmony*, 210).

25. Though she does admit that the abduction is an undeserved punishment, Irigaray goes so far as to chide Kore for picking flowers at all, as if she were offending the earth

by doing so. See Irigaray, *Thinking the Difference*, 102. Perhaps, picking flowers in a French garden would be inappropriate, but gardeners in America and Britain are familiar with those vast swaths of yellow flowers that appear in spring, blooming "like a crocus" across a "wide" landscape. Anyone who has enjoyed the dazzling profusion of spring bulbs knows that there are scenes in which one can pick flowers without leaving a trace. Such was the floriferous beauty of the plain of Nysa.

26. Pausanias, *Description of Greece*, 9.31.7–9.

27. See Irigaray, *Sexes and Genealogies*, on the impossibility of sustaining the mother/daughter relation under "the patriarchal regime," an impossibility that is "reinforced" by psychoanalysis (2). See also Irigaray, *I Love to You*, 26. This "erasure" of the relation between mother and daughter belongs to the installation of man as the "universal." It results in "the most extreme loss of human singularity . . . it can entail the end of the human species sacrificed to an abstract universal, absolute spirit."

28. Foley, *The Homeric Hymn to Demeter*, ll. 333, 339. Demeter, as generativity, cannot cross over into the underworld herself. She would be stuck forever with someone else's word.

29. Nonnus, *Dionysiaca*, 5.586–621. Zeus' ocular violence reappears, somewhat internalized and domesticated, in Rousseau's governor, who could not resist undressing the chastely dressed young girl in his imagination, item by item.

30. While Zeus and his brother put around the lie that Tantalus made a stew of his son and tried to feed it to the gods, Pindar confirms the truth. Poseidon lusted after the boy and abducted him. Demeter rescues him. Zeus condemns Tantalus to his gruesome punishment both for trying to share ambrosia with humans and as a cover story for Poseidon's crime. Pindar, *Olympian Ode*, 1.37–63.

31. Hades appears only on the battlefield to collect the dead. His other liaisons are with underground nymphs. Oppian describes Mintho as a "maid beneath the earth," while Leuce belongs to subterranean springs.

32. Diodorus Siculus, *Library of History*, 4.4.1 and 5.75.4.

33. Like Mukhtaran Mai's body, Pasiphae's body is a battleground in a dispute between male powers. Because Poseidon wishes to punish her husband Minos, who kept for himself the beautiful white bull owed to the god, Pasiphae is transformed from a great queen into a grotesque zoophiliac and the mother of a monster who dines on human flesh.

34. Rilke, *Duino Elegies*, ll. 76–83.

35. See Proust, *À la recherche du temps perdu*, 3:1037–38. Hegel describes life as a "highway of despair" because humans are always discovering that they are not who they thought they were.

36. Irigaray undervalues Demeter's power: "The only right to oppose this separation of mother and daughter is the right to bring sterility to the earth." But this is the right of life itself, the inversion of the infinite profusion of bodies (Irigaray, *Sexes and Genealogies*, 131).

37. Site officiel du musée du Louvre.

38. Across the room, in vitrine 4, is a second small statuette of two seated figures who may also be Demeter and Persephone, resting after a long day.

39. For centuries, women have been vulnerable to sexual violence, and their bodies have been treated as the property of men, to be disposed of at the convenience and judgment of men. The systematic rape of the enemy's women has regularly been a feature of war. Women are still raped or stoned to settle disputes among men or sacrificed, either by being killed or by being forcibly married. Today, in many parts of the world, girls as young as twelve or thirteen are sold into marriage or other forms of sexual service by their patriarchal masters. In the United States, girls and women are subject to the interference of the state and the church in their most intimate decisions about reproduction and effectively denied access to basic reproductive services due to strictures imposed by Congress. The U.S.'s infamous gag rule, which effectively defunded any aid organization that apprised women and girls of their full medical options, cost millions of lives. In New Delhi and many other large cities, women cannot go out alone without fear of harassment and are consequently not only subject to an environment of threat and violence but also to limitations on their mobility and agency that undermine their liberty and opportunity. See, e.g., http://www.unicef.org/infobycountry/india_70237.

40. The term *human being* suggests that humans exist in a way essentially different from other animals. The term *person* belongs to the rights of man. I employ the term *human-body* for mortals in order to emphasize the continuity of their being with other animals, to remark their essential embodiment, as over against the opposition of speculative reason to the body, and to grant mortals an existence outside the logic of property.

41. "Life itself" refers to no metaphysical entity, but to the becoming of all that comes into being, grows, and dies. "Life itself": the growing beings that once were not and will again not be. "Life itself": differentiated becoming in its richness and specificity. "Life itself": species thought as generations of individuals, a wild profusion of breathing, pulsing, morphing bodies. "Life itself": becoming and all of its artifacts. Stories, tools, houses: life itself. See Huffer, "Foucault's Fossils." Huffer presents a challenging critique of the attempt to base ethics and politics on a concept of life. "Life" thought beginning from the generativity of the two mothers is something "real" as in the thought of "renaturalizers," but not an ahistorical biological concept. On the other hand, it incorporates the elements of risk and fragility emphasized by "denaturalizers" without subscribing to a generic vitalism or pansexuality. It avoids the metaphysical turn and anthropomorphism that Huffer diagnoses not only by thinking life as life/death (birth, growth, metamorphosis, and death) but also by insisting on life itself as a claim. It cries out, like an infant, or a woman in pain, or a cheering crowd. The management and disposition of life under biopower, so familiar as to be almost invisible, must be made strange to attend to the claim of these cries.

Elizabeth Grosz demonstrates Darwin's reconceptualization of life as "fundamental becoming." "Life exceeds itself, its past, its context in making itself more and other than its history: life is that which registers and harnesses the impact of contingency, converting contingency into history, and history into self-overcoming, supercession, becoming-other" (Grosz, *Time Travels*, 40). This emphasis on the openness and futurity of life belongs to critical phenomenology too. Like Grosz, critical phenomenology links "this concept of a dynamized, uncontainable, unpredictable life: a life always lived in excess of need, in variation form its past and its antecedents and beyond any containment or systematicity" to "reconfiguring how we may understand social, political, cultural, and subjective relations" (42).

42. The widely circulated tale of the pomegranate is yet another example of the brothers' rumormongering to hide the agency and collaboration of the two mothers. It is implausible that so keenly perceptive and highly vigilant a creature as Persephone, after so much patience, would have, in haste, inadvertently eaten a few seeds, altering her destiny forever. She eats the seeds of her own volition, as a mark of her commitment to the logic of life/death and the linear time of mortals. The explosive fecundity of the pomegranate yields an abundance of life, and its deep red juice stains like the blood of life. Persephone, goddess of life/death, embraces it as her talisman, the emblem of her guardianship of mortals.

43. Kerényi, *Eleusis*, 148.

44. Irigaray notes the "risk" that is incurred in associating women with nature: "Women are the guardians of singularity, of a sensible understanding which is opposed to abstract extension. Unfortunately, their qualities are still considered as being bound only to nature, to matter, a situation which carries with it the risk of again falling away from the intellect and into immediate sensibility" (*To Be Two*, 72). The figure of Demeter and Persephone refigures this continuity with nature. Neither nature nor the female humanbody is a resource to be mastered and managed by man. Nature, life, and the elements of life command attentive and strategic labor. Demeter and Persephone figure this collaboration on behalf of the future and the conditions of life. Agriculture introduces transcendence, both the transcendence of immediacy in the deferral of desire and the transcendence of solitude in collective action.

45. Irigaray, *Democracy Begins Between Two*: "Humanity, particularly industrial capitalism, has put the planet itself in danger and there will not be a future unless we make the salvation of the earth itself our immediate concern. . . . Such an objective seems to me, today, to be the first one that we should pursue to ensure for each man and woman at least the right to life: to air, to water, to light, to the heat of the sun, to the nourishment of earth. Rescuing the planet Earth means, too, being concerned about happiness, as much for ourselves as others" (168). Irigaray links the "failure of respect for nature" to the subjection of women's generativity to "the geneaology of the husband," which is to say to the law of property. See *Sexes and Genealogies*, 3.

46. Hobbes, *Leviathan*, chapter 24, 170.

III: LIVABLE FUTURES

1. See Willett, *Interspecies Ethics*; Marder, *Plant-Thinking*.

2. Foucault, "Sex, Power, and the Politics of Identity," 172.

5. EATING AT THE HEART OF ETHICS

1. Aeschylus, *Prometheus Bound*, ll. 1025–26.
2. Poseidon, ever rapacious and resentful, abducted the youth Pelops, who had excited his lust. Zeus started the rumor of Pelops' dismemberment, both to provide a cover story for his disappearance and to justify the extreme punishment he had meted out to Tantalus for sharing ambrosia with humans. Pindar, *Olympian Ode*, 1l. 37–63; Apollodorus, *Library of Greek Mythology*, 12.2.1.
3. Rilke, *Duino Elegies*, ll. 76–83.
4. Shiva, *Staying Alive*, 121. See also, Montanari, *Food Is Culture*: "Indeed, scholars are pretty well in agreement in acknowledging a *female* priority in the work of observation and selection of plants that accompanied the birth of agriculture around the first village settlements" (7).
5. A chicken farmer needs only one rooster, a dairyman only one bull.
6. "Agribusiness" refers to an industrialized agriculture that seeks "vertical integration" or to control food from the point of production to the point of ingestion. It depends on nonrenewable inputs such as fertilizers, weed killers, and pesticides. It maximizes profits by inserting "processing" between staple food and the consumer. See, e.g., the World Bank's analysis of the way in which agriculture's ability to reduce poverty depends on the poor "connecting" to the key drivers of "growth," i.e., the shift to diets high in processed foods and "livestock products." World Bank, *Agriculture for Development*, 36–37. As Vandana Shiva points out, the World Bank and global agribusiness "reduce all value to market value and register only those activities and processes that are monetized" (*Staying Alive*, 220). Unfortunately, as Shiva notes "what is a 'value added' process [for agribusiness] is a 'value annihilation' process from the point of view of nutrition" (173).
7. Denton, "Climate Change Vulnerability."
8. https://sustainabledevelopment.un.org/content/documents/escap_doc.pdf. Her comment was made at the "Women Major Side Event" and appears as the epigraph to the report of that meeting. Document CSD16, UN Commission on Sustainable Development.
9. See, e.g., Nussbaum, *Women and Human Development*; Amartya Sen, "Women's Agency and Social Change," in *Development as Freedom*.
10. See, e.g., World Bank, "World Bank Group Agriculture Action Plan, FY 2010–12," 20ff. See also "Monsanto 2012 Annual Report," 30ff.
11. The American policy of giving food aid in surplus food artificially depresses prices and undermines the economic viability of the local farmer.
12. See, e.g., Forum for Food Sovereignty, "The Declaration of Nyéléni" (2007), signed by eight hundred representatives of eighty countries to assert the food sovereignty of local producers against "markets and corporations," or the documents and activities of Via Campesina, an international organization defending the rights of indigenous farmers and local food sovereignty (http://www.viacampesina.org).

13. See Nestle, *Food Politics*, 360.

14. Mill, *On Liberty*, 106–8.

15. Ibid.

16. Ibid.

17. Ismene, at liberty, "ran around" on behalf of her family, negotiating among conflicting powers to restore sociality. Her liberty was displayed not only in her physical mobility but also in her mobility of thought and feeling. Always ready to forgive, Ismene alone among the Cadmeans shows the fluidity, as opposed to hardness of heart and head, that is necessary to move forward. Liberty is nothing so thin and insubstantial as the choice to eat a Big Mac or not.

18. See Pollan's discussion of the history of policies in the United States favoring bigger farms. Pollan, *The Omnivore's Dilemma*, 48–53.

19. Leibniz, *Monadology*, paragraph #58.

20. Charles Francis et al., "Food Webs and Food Sovereignty." See also Pollan, *The Omnivore's Dilemma*, on the higher productivity of smaller over larger farms (161). In the twenty-first century, hunger derives from violence and climate disaster rather than poor farming techniques.

21. ETC Group, "New Report on Corporate Power" (http://www.etcgroup.org). See also Shiva, "The Seeds of Suicide." Also Sridhar, "Why Do Farmers Commit Suicide?"

22. See, e.g., Stein, "Intellectual Property and Genetically Modified Seeds." See also "Why Does Monsanto Sue Farmers Who Save Seeds?"

23. Rudel et al., "Changing Drivers of Deforestation."

24. Cf. President Obama's New Alliance for Food Security: this policy delivers the developing world to global agribusiness just as its markets in the developed world are declining (http://www.usaid.gov/unga/new-alliance).

25. Lang and Millstone, *The Atlas of Food*, 58–59.

26. Gottlieb and Joshi, *Food Justice*, 33.

27. Irigaray, *Sexes and Genealogies*, 127; see also her *An Ethics of Sexual Difference*, 126–29.

28. Pollan, *The Omnivore's Dilemma*, 73. Pollan is referring specifically to commodity corn.

29. See Pollan's discussion of the historic importance of the discovery of the Haber-Bosch process that made modern fertilizers possible, possibly the "most important invention of the twentieth century." It may have produced the fertilizer that prevented famine in China in the 1970s, but it has also "changed the earth's ecology" in ways that now threaten the generativity of earth itself (ibid., 41–47).

30. Agriculture contributes somewhere between 17 and 32 percent of greenhouse gases, much of that associated with the mechanization, inputs, and scale of agribusiness. Agribusiness adds the cost of transport, processing, and packaging as well, further increasing its contribution to global warming. See Lang and Millstone, *The Atlas of Food*, 63.

31. On the link between global food, obesity, and environmental degradation, see Alleyne et al., "Embedding Non-communicable Diseases."

32. So-called ag gag laws have been passed in several U.S. states criminalizing investigative reporting and whistleblowing on factory farms. See Schatz, "A War on Freedom and Food."

33. President Obama's 2013 New Alliance for Food Security is a case in point. While acknowledging the need to support indigenous farmers, particularly women, the policy and process do not include their voices. They do not have a seat at the table where decisions about their futures are being made.

34. See the discussion of labor practices in Gottlieb and Joshi, *Food Justice*, 37, 50, 54. See also McMillan, *The American Way of Eating*, which details the impossibility of eating well on the income of a food-industry worker.

35. See, e.g., United Nations Industrial Development Organization, "Fighting Poverty by Fostering Agro-value Chains."

36. Patel, *Stuffed and Starved*, 302.

37. Shiva, *Staying Alive*, xxiii.

38. Montanari, *Food Is Culture*, 33.

39. Ibid., 29. See also Lévi-Strauss, *The Raw and the Cooked*, on the link between cooking and being "socialized" (336). In certain cultures, menstruating or postpartum women must be "cooked" as a means of resocializing them after being "deeply involved in a physiological process."

40. Quoted in Gottlieb and Joshi, *Food Justice*, 60.

41. Despite the juggernaut of agribusiness and global food, the specificity of taste appears to be irreducible. See Montanari's discussion of the local variations that McDonald's has found it necessary to make in its standard menu (*Food Is Culture*, 85, 88–89).

42. Gortmacher et al., "Changing the Future of Obesity." See also Swinburn et al., "The Global Obesity Pandemic."

43. http://www.who.int/mediacentre/factsheets/fs311/en/.

44. Soekirman, "Taking the Indonesian Nutrition History," 448.

45. Atmarita, "Nutritional Problems in Indonesia."

46. Hawkes, "Uneven Dietary Development."

47. While utilitarianism may not rely directly on this myth, it does depend on a calculation of goods that arrays disparate values on a single scale, privileging "higher" social and cultural values over the values and interests of nature and the body that must eat or be eaten.

48. Pollan, *The Omnivore's Dilemma*, 84.

49. See Pollan's discussion of the ethics of eating meat (ibid., 307–13). See also Mason and Singer, *The Ethics of What We Eat*. Singer and others who insist on vegetarianism do not sufficiently regard the interdependence of domesticated animals and humans, nor do they accord sufficient weight to the costs to cultures, knowledges, and forms of life that a universal vegetarianism would exact.

50. This landscape, along with Jim Crow, has almost disappeared. It reflected the gender division of labor and racial segregation of the time. Every white Southerner who grew

up under Jim Crow remembers both the joy of a community entirely mediated by food and the familiar horrors of segregation. Only a stone is innocent.

51. Montanari, *Food Is Culture*, 17.

52. Quoted ibid., 15.

53. Ibid.

54. See Montanari's discussion of the link between dietetics and medicine's humoral theory. Appetite marks an imbalance of humors that can be addressed by the desired food (ibid., 51–57).

55. Ibid., 62.

56. The recent case of the celebrity chef Paula Deen would argue otherwise. http://abcnews.go.com/blogs/entertainment/celebrities/.

57. Marion Nestle reports that more is spent to advertise a single candy bar or soda "by a factor of 50 to 100" than is spent in a year by the educational program of the National Cancer Institute's "5 A Day" partnership with industry to promote consumption of five servings of fruits and vegetables daily (*Food Politics*, 369). See also Nestle's discussion of the strategies used by industry to capture school-age children as a market (ibid., 175–96).

58. Montanari, *Food Is Culture*, 94.

59. Ibid., 133.

60. See ibid., 62, where Montanari distinguishes *sapere* and *sapore*.

61. Proust, *À la recherche du temps perdu*, 1:43–48.

62. Boutonnat, *Au Coeur de la France*, 3.

63. Since Napoleon, the law of partible inheritance has required the division of estates among all heirs. This has led to a complex pattern of ownership in which a single vineyard may be owned by dozens of producers, who each may own only a row or two of vines. Unlike Bordeaux, which is dominated by large global corporate interests, Burgundy is still overwhelmingly in the hands of local families.

64. Boutonnat, *Au Coeur de la France*.

65. Le Grand Prix de la Baguette de la Ville de Paris.

66. Montanari errs in contrasting the regionalism of Italy with the centralization of France. The latter facilitates a regionalism that is no less distinct and differentiated than in Italy. It is precisely this combination of a thoroughgoing centralization of human affairs with an intense regionalism that is distinctively French. See Montanari, *Food Is Culture*, 79.

67. As de Gaulle remarked, "Comment voulez-vous gouverner un pays qui a deux cent quarante-six variétés de fromage?" (Mignon, *Les mots du general*). While the governing region has no cheeses of its own, it protects and preserves the distinction of each region.

68. Boutonnat, *Au Coeur de la France*.

69. La Fédération des fromagers de France claims over a thousand distinct French cheeses. www.fromagersdefrance.com.

70. Rozin et al., "The Ecology of Eating: Smaller Portion Sizes in France."
71. Recent research has sought to debunk the "French paradox," but disparities in diet, eating habits, and health outcomes still tend to favor the French model. See Law and Wald, "Why Heart Disease Mortality Is Low in France." But see also the commentary on this article by D. J. P. Barker.
72. Taste Jason Atherton's delicious riff on this aspect of rural cooking: Head to Toe, Pollen Street Social, Pollen Street, London.

6. A WORKING LIFE

1. Hobbes, *Leviathan*, 63.
2. A recent *New York Times* article detailing the toll taken on a single mother by these labor practices resulted in efforts at policy change by the employer. See Kantor, "Working Anything But 9 to 5" and "Starbucks to Revise Policies."
3. Roosevelt, "The 'Four Freedoms' Speech."
4. Hobbes, *Leviathan*, 88–89.
5. Roosevelt, "First Inaugural Address."
6. Pollan, *The Omnivore's Dilemma*, 244–45.
7. Paulson, "Ag-gag Bills Harm Free Speech." On the environmental harm posed by CAFOs, see Gottlieb and Joshi, *Food Justice*, 33.
8. Hobbes, *Leviathan*, 174.
9. Wolff, *The Asset Price Meltdown*.
10. "When the global trend is isolated, we find that, in the last two decades, inequality has increased throughout the world in a pattern that cuts across the effect of national income changes. During the decades that happen to coincide with the rise of neoliberal ideology, with the breakdown of national sovereignties, and with the end of Keynesian policies in the global debt crisis of the early 1980s, inequality rose worldwide." Galbraith, "A Perfect Crime."
11. Nussbaum, *Women and Human Development*, 65. See also Baudrillard, *The Consumer Society*, 41–42.
12. Sen, "The Concept of Development," 161–62.
13. China is currently experiencing a forced "urbanization" as the government pursues a policy of displacing rural farmers in an effort to turn them into urban consumers. See, e.g., Johnson, "China's Great Uprooting." Large-scale global projects like dams regularly require the displacement of local peoples. See, e.g., Asthana, "Forced Displacement." During the 1990s, about 10 million people a year globally were displaced by development projects. See Cernea, "The Risks and Reconstruction Model for Resettling Displaced Populations."
14. Shiva, *Earth Democracy*, 130.
15. U.S. president Barack Obama's recent 3 billion dollar deal with agribusiness to "develop" agriculture in developing nations is a case in point. While paying lip service to small, indigenous farmers, the agreement clearly paves the way for their displacement

by global capital. They do not have a seat at the table in the discussions that determine their future. See Rawlinson, "Obama and Agribusiness."

16. See, for example, Amartya Sen's discussion of how the systematic deprivation of girls in some communities escapes income analysis or the way in which, in Anglo-European countries, women's labor is "unrecognized." Sen, *Development as Freedom*, 88–89. See note 8, 320, for an extensive bibliography on the undervaluing and invisibility of women's labor under the development strategies of global capital. See also 115 where Sen articulates "the freedom of women to seek employment outside the family." Sen, like Irigaray, argues that the exercise of this free will requires significant reconfigurations in the family. Like Foucault, Sen argues that the exercise of this freedom will disturb "prevailing perceptions of 'normality' and 'appropriateness.'"

17. See Irigaray, "Ten Suggestions for the Construction of the European Union":

> Often the help which we plan to give to less wealthy countries is a way of imposing industrialization as we know it on them. . . . We know what the relationship between industrialization, capitalism, and slavery is. We also know what the limits of industrialization are as regards employment, yet we go on involving other countries in this process and, in this way, win a few more years for an economic regime whose blind alleys should be all too obvious to us.
>
> In my view, it would be fairer politically-speaking to encourage a form of economic development that was appropriate to the environment and culture of a country, in other words to promote economic diversity rather than imposing a single and inevitably competitive model.
>
> (IBID., 159)

18. Ehrenreich, *Nickled and Dimed*; McMillan, *The American Way of Eating*.

19. While the difficulty in obtaining reliable data is regularly cited, most sources suggest that the victims of human trafficking number in the millions annually. The UNODC report on human trafficking estimates that, of the two to four million cases annually, 80 percent involve sexual exploitation, overwhelmingly of women and girls. See United Nations Office on Drugs and Crime, "Global Report on Trafficking in Persons."

20. A recent study of the "Gilgo Girls," a series of prostitutes abducted, murdered, and buried on a Long Island beach, reveals how these working-class women were driven to work as "escorts" because of the impossibility of actually supporting themselves and their children on the low-wage service jobs to which they had access. See Kolker, *Lost Girls*.

21. Hossain, "Rana Plaza Collapse Victims."

22. See, e.g., Urbina, "Buying Overseas Clothing." The article surveys working conditions at various garment factories in Central America and Asia.

23. Plato, *Republic*, 370c, 433a.

24. Ibid., 350b.

25. Demeter will have nothing less than the living presence of her daughter, Persephone, "looking back."

26. Nussbaum, *Women and Human Development*, 117, note 7. Plato may not relegate experience to quite so low a philosophical role as Platonism would have it, but his commitment to vertical authority seems undeniable.

27. Roosevelt, "The 'Four Freedoms' Speech."

28. Eisenhower, "The Military-Industrial Complex Speech."

29. Spiraling health care costs in the United States cannot and should not be addressed by cutting benefits. What is not sustainable is the fee-for-service delivery of medical care or the profits of the insurance industry. The delivery of care needs to be reorganized around patients, not procedures. Medicare has been significantly more efficient and cost effective than private insurers and should be universalized.

30. In the time of the twenty-first century's Great Recession, this must be amended to *actual* callous and selfish wrongdoing by banks and global financial institutions.

31. Roosevelt, "First Inaugural Address."

32. Kocieniewski. "A Shuffle of Aluminum"; *New York Times* editorial board, "Goldman Sachs Aluminum Pile."

33. Vandana Shiva demonstrates how the supposedly "higher yields" of the Green Revolution "disappear in the context of total yields of crops on farms." Higher yields of wheat or maize were achieved at the expense of straw. Resulting reductions in fodder amounted to "stealing food from animals and soil organisms." See Shiva, *Stolen Harvest*, 12.

34. In 2013, multiple women complained that the mayor of San Diego was an abusive employer who indulged in various forms of sexual harassment. A total of seventeen complaints were made against him, and, after initially refusing to resign, he was forced out of office in August 2013. At his resignation, he protested his innocence and decried the "lynch mob" that had attacked him. Two months later, he pled guilty to charges of battery and false imprisonment involving three women. The celebrity cook Paula Deen, who built a multimillion dollar empire on Southern food, has recently been exposed for her indulgence in racist attitudes and for her failure to share her success with the black employees on whom her business depended. While these are famous cases, the attitudes of these employers are unfortunately all too common in the workplace.

35. Kemp, "Iowa Court OKs Firing of Female Dental Assistant."

36. Bergman, "Rape in the Fields."

37. In the United States in the last quarter century, education has been corrupted by political ideologies of "accountability." Of course, accountability and assessment are important in education, but the primary result of this ideological approach has been the explosion of a testing industry that commands an ever greater share of funding, time, and focus in education. At the same time, a parallel track of "charter" schools has developed, which are largely publicly funded, but able to establish criteria of admission, siphoning resources, personnel, and space from open admission schools. Experts agree that the one thing that improves student learning at all levels is smaller classes; yet policies do not focus on training, supporting, and rewarding teachers, but on identifying "bad" teachers. Failing students and schools tend to reflect larger socioeconomic

inequities beyond the classroom teacher's agency. Current policies drive the best teachers away from the most demanding schools. Nothing would improve student learning more and more quickly than ending all federal funding of testing and using the money to hire, train, and reward classroom teachers.

38. No one wants to be the young black American male of statistical probabilities: a 29 percent chance of spending time in prison, for example, compared with 4 percent for a white male. Black men are also more likely than whites or other racial groups to be the victims of violent crime. See U.S. Department of Justice, "Black Victims of Violent Crime." Identified by these statistics, a black man, anyone, would want to exercise the freedom (not) to be who he is. Anyone would insist on being otherwise—or rather on changing the conditions of identity to make it possible to be otherwise than these predictions.

39. Irigaray, *An Ethics of Sexual Difference*, 5.

40. Breen and Cook, "The Persistence of the Gendered Division of Labor."

41. Rosenthal, "American Way of Birth."

42. Reineke, "*In Vitro Veritas*."

43. In 2013 the French parliament was 18.5 percent women, while women held 18.5 percent of the seats in the U.S. House of Representatives and 20 percent in the Senate. In both states women held about 15 percent of seats on corporate boards. In both states women held about 30 percent of the positions in higher education, but less than 20 percent of full professorships and less than 10 percent of academic leadership positions.

44. Hersch, "Opting Out Among Women with Elite Education." See also Steiner, *Mommy Wars* and Lerner, *The War on Moms*.

45. Despite this toil and lack of luxury, no one could be more generous. A stranger walking a road through small farms and villages is repeatedly pressed to stop and share a chapati. The women admire my red nail polish, and I their bangles. Without sharing any language, we share this small encounter in which I am a curious but welcome interruption in their labors.

46. See www.dastkar.org.

47. For other concrete examples, see Kristof and WuDunn, *Half the Sky* and *A Path Appears*.

IV: SOVEREIGN BODIES

1. Contemporary writers like Fukuyama deeply misunderstand Hegel's claim about the "end of history." Hegel does not look forward to a terminal utopian moment, as Fukuyama claims; rather, he makes a logical or conceptual point. If "ours is a birthtime of Spirit," it is because all the possible shapes of human subjectivity and all the possible forms of objectivity have actually been realized in history, so that they are available for reflection and articulation as concepts. This does not relieve human beings of the necessity of making a life, nor of the role of contingency in history, nor of the vulnerability of human institutions to those contingencies. There is always, for Hegel, at least

the Hegel of the *Phenomenology of Spirit*, more to be done in the project of liberation and more work to be done to sustain the collaborations and reciprocities of genuine community. See Fukuyama, *The End of History and the Last Man*, xii; cf. Hegel, *Phenomenology of Spirit*, #11. Undoing Hegel's installation of the gender division of labor as a solution to the problem of nourishing both the world of needy bodies and familial relations, on the one hand, and the public work of science, politics, and philosophy, on the other, opens history to unheard-of possibilities.

2. Rilke, "The Ninth Elegy," in *Duino Elegies*, 65.

3. During the 1990s in the United States, the image of "welfare queens" drove a dismantling of welfare policy that forced many mothers of young children who were also students into the workforce. They were forced to give up their educations and futures in exchange for low-paying, dead-end jobs. Since then, the rhetoric of blaming the poor for their poverty and the unemployed for their lack of work has only become more virulent. At a recent meeting at the American Enterprise Institute, a conservative think tank, the speaker of the U.S. House of Representatives, John Boehner, stated that people have "this idea" that "I really don't have to work. I don't really want to do this. I think I'd rather just sit around" (quoted in Krugman, "Those Lazy Jobless"). The poor and unemployed are just lazy. The moral callus that allows politicians to abuse their own constituents in this way and to ignore the real suffering that the lack of adequate employment causes must be rubbed raw.

    Ironically, it was an additional federal program supporting families that can be credited for the gains in employment after welfare reform. "Regression results indicate that Temporary Assistance to Needy Families (TANF), the federal program created in 1996 pursuant to the welfare reform law, accounts for more than half of the decline in welfare participation and more than 60 percent of the rise in employment among single mothers." O'Neil and Hill, "Civic Report 17." Putting aside the question of what long-term effects will be suffered by the children, now entering adulthood, whose mothers were forced into work in the absence of any adequate child-care infrastructure, the authors' claims for the success of welfare reform now appear premature. In 2012 only twenty-five of every one hundred families in poverty received TANF. Since the Great Recession of 2007–2009, the value of its payments has eroded, while many states have made steep cuts in the program. Shift work or part-time work and widespread unemployment have left many families struggling or homeless. Pavetti and Schott, "TANF's Inadequate Response to the Recession."

4. The emergence of contemporary bioethics in the 1970s in the United States is framed by a concern about the harm done when the specificity of the patient is reduced to a general form or protocol. See, e.g., Ramsey, *The Patient as Person*. For accounts of the deleterious clinical effects of these abstractions and the abstract thinking that deploys them, see, e.g., Cassell, *The Healer's Art*. The recent advent of digitized protocols for taking the history and physical of a patient has not only undermined a crucial medical skill but also literally reduced the specificity of the patient's narrative to a general

form. While it is important to digitize medical records to protect data and make them accessible and shareable, the digitizing of the moment of intake has contributed to the tendency to reduce the patient to a preexisting category and to subject her to protocols that are not informed by the specificities of her existence.

5. "The other is from the first the brother to all men." Levinas, *Otherwise Than Being or Beyond Essence*, 158. See Simon Critchley's critique of Levinas' characterization of the feminine as the "pre-ethical opening of the ethical." Critchley, *The Ethics of Deconstruction*, 136–37.

6. Kant's moral subject, e.g., acts "as if" he belongs to a kingdom ends, "as if" his action followed a "universal law of nature" or were governed by the "idea" of autonomy. Kant, *Groundwork of the Metaphysics of Morals*, 106–7. See Hegel's critique of this "unhappy consciousness," a bifurcated living being who is promised resolution only after death. *Phenomenology of Spirit*, #207–30. Though the critique is directed at Christian theories of salvation and the practices associated with them, it also takes aim at the Kantian moral subject.

7. *Phenomenology of Spirit*, #430–31.

8. The UN and its human rights regimes consistently fail to hold member states accountable for the subjection of women in any meaningful way. No one is boycotting Saudi Arabia or treating it as an international pariah like apartheid South Africa. The regime of rights coexists with the subjection of women and is sustained by the same complex of forces. It exhibits no effective allergy to the current "collective structures" in spite of its declarations. To the extent that the heroic work of the UN's Section on Gender and many NGOs focuses on extending the rights of man to women, it remains complicit with the logic of fraternity and capital that sustains both rights and the subjection of women.

9. As this book goes to press, the U.S. National Football League, an American cultural monument, is embroiled in a scandal over its toleration of domestic abuse among star players. Barker, "Scandals Put the NFL in Congress's Crosshairs." While these scandals have brought attention to violence against women, the NFL has always used women to sell its product. See the scantily clad cheerleaders who accompany games at www.nfl.com/photos/0ap2000000281882. They function similarly to the models who are hired to decorate club openings and can expect a similar fate: low pay, injury, sexual predation, and a career that lasts only as long as their youth and looks. It is the male owners who reap the profits of their bodies and beauty.

10. Neither governments nor medicine can justify their complicity in these markets. Even the need for organs does not justify taking advantage of the social inequity that would lead someone to sell a kidney.

11. See Irigaray, *Democracy Begins Between Two*, 150–51.

12. See also Irigaray, *Sexes and Genealogies*, 132 and *Je, Tu, Nous*, 103 on "forced motherhood" as an "unbearable injustice."

13. Plato, *Republic*, 350b.

14. Aisch and Marsh, "How Likely Is It?"

15. Physicians who do not want to perform this service should find another line of work. Such a refusal is no more defensible in a physician than refusing, on religious grounds, to give a patient a blood transfusion.

16. In the United States abortion providers have regularly been subject to violence, and eight have been murdered. The physical separation of these services from other medical practices has made both patients and caregivers vulnerable to regular picketing and heckling. The antiabortion movement has also been successful in imposing restrictions that require the closure of many clinics in some states. The courts are currently debating whether a three- or four-hour drive to a clinic and a forty-eight-hour waiting period constitute an "undue burden" on a woman trying to exercise her constitutionally guaranteed right to manage her reproductive destiny.

17. Considerable research from the WHO, various UN agencies, private foundations, and scholars indicates that improving women's health, increasing women's economic independence, and educating girls are among the most efficient and effective interventions that can be made to improve the overall welfare of a community. These interventions assuage poverty and overpopulation, increase the general level of education, and reduce violent extremism, tribalism, and terrorism. For excellent summaries of this research see Kristof and WuDunn, *Half the Sky* and *A Path Appears*. The latter text gives many examples of programs that are successful in "shattering our current structures" to improve the future of communities by improving the agency of women. This future is no utopian dream.

18. The "advent or event of the other" elicits wonder. Irigaray, *An Ethics of Sexual Difference*, 75.

19. Georges Bataille, "The Love of Truth and Justice and the Socialism of Marcel Proust," in *Literature and Evil*, 145.

20. Potter, *Bioethics*.

21. Irigaray, *I Love to You*, 110.

22. Irigaray, *Democracy Begins Between Two*, 96.

23. Irigaray, *Sexes and Genealogies*, 4.

24. Irigaray, *Democracy Begins Between Two*, 167.

25. Michel Foucault, "The Masked Philosopher," in *Ethics*, 327.

26. Ibid., 325.

27. Foucault, *Ethics*, 172.

28. Irigaray, *Democracy Begins Between Two*, 159.

29. Ibid, 62.

30. Kant, "To Eternal Peace," 453.

31. Derrida, *The Beast and the Sovereign*, 1:272; quoting Kant, "Conjectures on the Beginnings of Human History."

32. After centuries of efforts to constrain it and contain it in the interlocked binaries of male/female–heterosexual/homosexual and to subdue it to the law of property, it is impossible to know what wonders may lie unthought in human sexuality. Perhaps the

best thing for philosophy and medicine, as well as commerce and advertising, is to say *nothing at all* about sex and sexuality. It is time for philosophy, medicine, science, and commerce to shut up for a while about sex and sexuality and to let life speak for itself. Perhaps Annares, the anarchic world of Ursula Le Guin's *The Dispossessed*, provides a model: states should prohibit the sexualization of children, so that they may discover their sexuality on their own, while providing contraception and letting polymorphism proliferate. Then there might be something to say about human sexuality, rather than about the codes and laws to which it has been subjected.

33. Conniff, "Useless Creatures."
34. Pepper Martin, www.dizzydean.com/.
35. In a book on the right to life, it has not been possible to do justice to the claim of the lithic. While humans are among those animals that cling to the surface of Earth, many creatures live happily beneath the ground, amid rock, stone, and dirt. The lithic may not be living, but it commands respect as an infrastructure of life. Life depends on the generativity of the soil that sustains the miracle of the seed. Moreover, the lithic itself commands respect as the embodiment of time and Earth's history.

Bibliography

Ackroyd, Peter. *London: A Biography*. Norwell, MA: Anchor, 2012.

Aeschylus. *Prometheus Bound*. Cambridge: Harvard University Press, 2006.

Agamben, Giorgio. *Homo Sacer: Sovereign Power and Bare Life*. Palo Alto, CA: Stanford University Press, 1995.

Aisch, Gregor and Bill Marsh. "How Likely Is It That Birth Control Could Let You Down?" *New York Times*, September 13, 2014.

Alleyne, George, Agnes Binagwaho, Andy Haines, Selim Jahan, Rachel Nugent, Ariella Rjhani, and David Stuckler. "Embedding Non-communicable Diseases in the Post-2015 Development Agenda." *Lancet* 381, no. 9866 (2013): 566–74.

"Antigone—Analysis of Major Characters." SparkNotes. Accessed October 31, 2014. http://www.sparknotes.com/drama/antigone/canalysis.html.

Apollodorus. *Library of Greek Mythology*. New York: Oxford University Press, 1997.

Asthana, Vandana. "Forced Displacement: A Gendered Analysis of the Tehri Dam Project." *Economic and Political Weekly* 47, nos. 47–48 (2012): 96–102.

Athanassakis, Apostolos N., and Benjamin M. Wolkow, trans. *The Orphic Hymns*. Baltimore: Johns Hopkins University Press, 2013.

Atmarita, Ita. "Nutritional Problems in Indonesia." Presentation given at the Integrated International Seminar on Life-Style Related Diseases. Gadjah Mada University. Yogyakarta, Indonesia. March 2005. http://gizi.depkes.go.id/download/nutrition%20problem%20in%20Indonesia.pdf.

Ballantyne, Angela. "Exploitation in Cross-Border Reproductive Care." *International Journal of Feminist Approaches to Bioethics* 7, no. 1 (Fall 2014): 75–99.

Barker, Jeff. "Scandals Put the NFL in Congress's Crosshairs." *Baltimore Sun*, September 21, 2014.

Barker-Benfield, G. J. *Horrors of the Half-Known Life*. New York: Harper and Row, 1976.

Bataille, Georges. *Literature and Evil*. Trans. Alistair Hamilton. New York: Penguin, 2012.

Baudrillard, Jean. *The Agony of Power.* Los Angeles: Semiotexte, 2010.

——. *Amérique.* Paris: Bernard Grasset, 1986.

——. *Carnival and Cannibal, or The Play of Global Antagonism.* Trans. Chris Turner. London: Seagull, 2010.

——. *The Consumer Society: Myths and Structures.* London: Sage, 1998 [1970].

——. "Ventriloquist Evil." In *Carnival and Cannibal, or The Play of Global Antagonism,* 31–92. Trans. Chris Turner. London: Seagull, 2010.

Benhabib, Seyla. *The Claims of Culture: Equality and Diversity in the Global Era.* Princeton: Princeton University Press, 2002.

——. "Multiculturalism and Gendered Citizenship." In *The Claims of Culture: Equality and Diversity in the Global Era,* 82–104. Princeton: Princeton University Press, 2002.

——. "On Hegel, Women, and Irony." In *Situating the Self: Gender, Community, and Postmodernism in Contemporary Ethics,* 242–59. New York: Routledge, 1992.

——. *Situating the Self: Gender, Community and Postmodernism in Contemporary Ethics.* New York: Routledge, 1992.

Bergman, Lowell. "Rape in the Fields." PBS *Frontline,* June 25, 2013.

Bianchi, Suzanne M. and Melissa A. Milke. "Work and Family Research in the First Decade of the Twenty-first Century." *Journal of Marriage and Family* 72, no. 3 (June 2010): 705–25. doi: 10.1111/j.1741–3737.2010.00726.x.

Blackstone, William. *Commentaries on the Laws of England.* Chicago: University of Chicago Press, 1979 [1765].

Borrelli-Persson, Laird. "Runway Review: Hervé Léger by Max Azria Spring 2009 Ready-to-Wear." *Style.com.* Last modified September 7, 2008. http://www.style.com/fashion-shows/spring-2009-ready-to-wear/herve-leger-by-max-azria.

Botterell, Andrew and Carolyn McLeod. "Can a Right to Reproduce Justify the Status Quo on Parental Licensing?" In *Permissible Progeny,* ed. S. Brennan et al. New York: Oxford University Press, forthcoming.

Boutonnat, Yves. *Au coeur de la France des 1000 fromages.* Tours: Ouest-France, 2003.

Breen, Richard, and Lynne Price Cook. "The Persistence of the Gendered Division of Labor." *European Sociological Review* 21, no. 1 (2005): 43–57.

Brillat-Savarin, Jean Anthelme. "Aphorism 4." In *The Physiology of Taste or Meditations on Transcendental Gastronomy,* 15. Trans. M. F. K. Fisher. New York: Knopf.

Brody, Elaine M. *Women in the Middle.* New York: Springer, 1990.

Buffett, Peter. "The Charitable-Industrial Complex." *New York Times,* July 26, 2013.

Butler, Judith. *Antigone's Claim.* New York: Columbia University Press, 1993.

——. *Gender Trouble.* New York: Routledge, 1990.

Calasso, Roberto. *The Marriage of Cadmus and Harmony.* New York: Vintage, 1994.

Campbell, Denis. "Models Reveal Why They Need a Union." *Guardian.* Last modified December 16, 2007. http://www.theguardian.com/uk/2007/dec/16/fashion.lifeand health.

Cassell, Eric. *The Healer's Art.* Cambridge: MIT Press, 1985.

Castillo, Michelle. "Women Undergoing Foot Surgery to Fit Into Heels Better." *CBS News.* Last modified November 28, 2012. http://www.cbsnews.com/news/women -undergoing-foot-surgery-to-fit-into-heels-better.

Cernea, Michael. "The Risks and Reconstruction Model for Resettling Displaced Populations." *World Development* 25, no. 10 (1997): 1569–87.

Chandler, Raymond. *The Simple Art of Murder.* New York: Vintage, 1988.

Chandler, Susan. "Revealing Look at Preteen Chic: Child Fashion Makes Some Uncomfortable." *Chicago Tribune,* August 30, 1998.

Charo, R. Alta. "The Endarkenment." In *The Ethics of Bioethics: Mapping the Moral Landscape,* ed. Lisa A. Eckenwiler and Felicia G. Cohn, 95–107. Baltimore: Johns Hopkins University Press, 2007.

Conniff, Richard. "Useless Creatures." *New York Times,* September 14, 2014.

Critchley, Simon. *The Ethics of Deconstruction.* Edinburgh: Edinburgh University Press, 1992.

Crozier, G. K. D., Jennifer L. Johnson, and Christopher Hajzler. "At the Intersections of Emotional and Biological Labor: Understanding Transnational Commercial Surrogacy as Social Reproduction." *International Journal of Feminist Approaches to Bioethics* 7, no. 2 (Fall 2014): 45–74.

Cruz, Julie. "Adidas Targets Teenage Girls for 1.3 Billion in Sales." *Bloomberg News,* March 19, 2013.

Cunningham, Bill. "On the Street: Catwalk." *New York Times,* September 13, 2009.

Curran, Bronwyn. "Mukhtaran Mai: The Other Side of the Story." *International News.* Last modified April 30, 2011. http://www.thenews.com.pk/Todays-News-9-44406 -Mukhtaran-Mai-the-other-side-of-the-story.

Cutler, David M., Edward L. Glaeser, and Jesse M. Shapiro, "Why Have Americans Become More Obese?" *Journal of Economic Perspectives* 17, no. 3 (2003): 93–118.

DeBruin, Debra A. "Ethics on the Inside?" In *The Ethics of Bioethics: Mapping the Moral Landscape,* ed. Lisa A. Eckenwiler, and Felicia G. Cohn, 161–69. Baltimore: Johns Hopkins University Press, 2007.

The Declaration of Independence. In *A Documentary History of the United States*, ed. Richard D. Heffner, 15–19. New York: Signet, 1965.

Denton, Fatma. "Climate Change Vulnerability, Impacts, and Adaptations: Why Does Gender Matter?" *Gender and Development* 10, no. 2 (2002): 10–20.

Derrida, Jacques. *The Beast and the Sovereign*, vol. 1. Trans. Geoffrey Bennington. Chicago: University of Chicago Press, 2009.

———. "Différance." In *Margins of Philosophy*, 1–27. Trans. Alan Bass. Chicago: University of Chicago Press, 1982.

———. "From Restricted to General Economy: An Hegelianism Without Reserve." In *Writing and Difference,* 251–77. Trans. Alan Bass. Chicago: University of Chicago Press, 1978.

———. *Margins of Philosophy.* Trans. Alan Bass. Chicago: University of Chicago Press, 1982.

———. *Speech and Phenomena.* Trans. David B. Allison. Evanston, IL: Northwestern University Press, 1973.

———. *Writing and Difference*. Trans. Alan Bass. Chicago: University of Chicago Press, 1978.

Diodorus Siculus. *Library of History*. 12 vols. Trans. C. H. Oldfather et al. Cambridge: Harvard University Press, 1933–1967.

"Dress Code Debate Heats Up Around the Country." ABC News. Last modified June 16, 2014. http://abcnews.go.com/GMA/video/dress-code-debate-heats-country-24153532.

Duffy, John. "Masturbation and Clitoridectomy: A Nineteenth-Century View." *Journal of the American Medical Association* 186, no. 3 (October 1963): 246–48.

Durisin, Megan. "12 Sexed-Up Brands That Market to Teens." *Business Insider,* March 19, 2013.

Ehrenreich, Barbara. *Nickel and Dimed: On (Not) Getting By in America*. New York: Holt, 2001.

Ehrenreich, Barbara and Deirdre English. *Complaints and Disorders: The Sexual Politics of Sickness*. Old Westbury, NY: Feminist Press, 1973.

Eisenhower, Dwight D. "The Military-Industrial Complex Speech." In *Public Papers of the Presidents: Dwight D. Eisenhower (1953–1961)*, 8 vols., 8:1035–40. Washington, DC: United States Government Printing Office, 1999.

Engelhardt, H. T. "The Disease of Masturbation." *Bulletin of the History of Medicine* 48, no. 2 (Summer 1974): 234–48.

Esteva, Gustavo. Address to the Conference of the Society for International Development. Rome, 1985.

ETC Group. "New Report on Corporate Power—Oligopoly, Inc. 2005." Last modified December 16, 2005. http://www.etcgroup.org/content/new-report-corporate-power-oligopoly-inc-2005.

Evans, Tony. *The Politics of Human Rights*. London: Pluto, 2005.

Executive Suite. Robert Wise, director. MGM, 1954.

Folbre, Nancy. *Valuing Children: Rethinking the Economics of the Family*. Cambridge: Harvard University Press, 2010.

Foley, Helen, ed. and trans. *The Homeric Hymn to Demeter*. Princeton: Princeton University Press, 1994.

Forum for Food Sovereignty. "The Declaration of Nyéléni." Nyeleni 2007. Last modified February 27, 2007. http://nyeleni.org/spip.php?article290.

Foucault, Michel. *Abnormal: Lectures at the Collège de France 1974–75*. Trans. Graham Burchell. New York: Picador, 2003.

———. *The Birth of Biopolitics: Lectures at the Collège de France 1978–79*. Trans. Graham Burchell. New York: Picador, 2008.

———. *The Birth of the Clinic: An Archaeology of Medical Perception*. Trans. A. M. Sheridan Smith. New York: Random House, 1973.

———. *Discipline and Punish: The Birth of the Prison*. Trans. Alan Sheridan. New York: Vintage, 1979.

———. *Ethics: Subjectivity and Truth*. New York: New Press, 1997.

———. *The Hermeneutics of the Subject: Lectures at the Collège de France 1981–1982*. Trans. Graham Burchell. New York: Picador, 2005.

———. *The History of Sexuality*, vol. 1. Trans. Robert Hurley. New York: Random House, 1978.

———. "The Masked Philosopher." In *Ethics: Subjectivity and Truth*, 321–28. New York: New Press, 1997.

———. "On the Genealogy of Ethics." In *Ethics: Subjectivity and Truth*. New York: New Press, 1997.

———. *The Order of Things*. New York: Vintage, 1973.

———. *Security, Territory, Population: Lectures at the Collège de France 1977–1978*. Trans. Graham Burchell. New York: Picador, 2009.

———. "Sex, Power, and the Politics of Identity." In *Ethics: Subjectivity and Truth*, 165–74. New York: New Press, 1997.

———. "The Social Triumph of the Sexual Will." In *Ethics: Subjectivity and Truth*, 157–64. New York: New Press, 1997.

———. *Society Must Be Defended: Lectures at the Collège de France 1975–1976*. Trans. David Macey. New York: Picador, 2003.

———. "Subjectivity and Truth." In *Ethics: Subjectivity and Truth*, 87–92. New York: New Press, 1997.

———. "What Is Enlightenment?" In *Ethics: Subjectivity and Truth*, 303–20. New York: New Press, 1997.

Francis, Charles, et al. "Food Webs and Food Sovereignty: Research Agenda for Sustainability." *Journal of Agriculture, Food Systems, and Community Development* 3, no. 4 (2003): 1–7.

Freud, Sigmund. *Civilization and Its Discontents*. In *The Standard Edition of the Complete Psychological Works of Sigmund Freud*, 21:57–145. Trans. James Strachey. London: Hogarth, 1961.

———. *Introductory Lectures on Psychoanalysis*. In *The Standard Edition of the Complete Psychological Works of Sigmund Freud*, 16:320–38. Trans. James Strachey. London: Hogarth, 1961.

Fukuyama, Francis. *The End of History and the Last Man*. New York: Avon, 1992.

Galbraith, James K. "A Perfect Crime: Global Inequality." *Daedalus* 131, no. 2 (2002): 11–25.

Galtung, Johan. *Human Rights in Another Key*. Cambridge: Polity, 1994.

Gilman, Charlotte Perkins. *The Yellow Wallpaper*. London: Penguin, 2009.

Gortmacher, Stephen L., David Levy, Rob Carter, Patricia L. Mabry, Diane T. Finegood, Terry Huang, Tim Marsh, and Marjory L. Moody. "Changing the Future of Obesity: Science, Policy, and Action." *Lancet* 37, no. 9793 (2011): 838–47.

Gottlieb, Robert and Anupama Joshi. *Food Justice*. Cambridge: MIT Press, 2010.

Government of India, Ministry of Health and Family Welfare. *National Guidelines for Accreditation, Supervision and Regulation of ART Clinics in India*. New Delhi: National Academy of Medical Sciences, 2005.

Groneman, Carol. "The Historical Construction of Female Sexuality." *Signs: Journal of Women in Culture and Society* 19, no. 2 (Winter 1993–4): 1–32.

Grosz, Elizabeth. *Time Travels: Feminism, Nature, Power.* Durham, NC: Duke University Press, 2005.

Gupta, Jyotsna A. "Reproductive Biocrossings: Indian Egg Donors and Surrogates in the Globalized Fertility Market." *International Journal of Feminist Approaches to Bioethics* 5, no. 1 (Spring 2012): 25–51.

Gutiérrez, Gustavo. *The Power of the Poor in History.* Trans. Robert R. Barr. Eugene, OR: Wipf and Stock, 2004.

Hausmann, Ricardo, Laura D. Tyson, and Saadia Zahidi. "The Global Gender Gap Report 2012." World Economic Forum. Accessed November 1, 2014. http://www3.weforum.org/docs/WEF_GenderGap_Report_2012.pdf.

Hawkes, Corinna. "Uneven Dietary Development: Linking the Policies and Processes of Globalization with the Nutrition Transition, Obesity, and Diet-Related Chronic Diseases." *Globalization and Health* 2, no. 4 (2006). doi: 10.1186/17440-8603-2-4.

Hegel, G. W. F. *Phenomenology of Spirit.* Trans. A. V. Miller. New York: Oxford University Press, 1977 [1807].

——. *Elements of the Philosophy of Right.* Trans. Allen Wood. New York: Cambridge University Press, 1991.

Heidegger, Martin. *Being and Time.* Trans. John Macquarrie and Edward Robinson. New York: Harper and Row, 1962.

Herndl, Diane Price. *Invalid Women: Figuring Feminine Illness in American Fiction and Culture, 1840–1940.* Chapel Hill: University of North Carolina Press, 1993.

Hersch, Joni. "Opting Out Among Women with Elite Education." *Social Science Research Network.* Vanderbilt Law and Economics Research Paper No. 13–5. April 24, 2013.

Hesiod. *Theogony.* Trans. Apostolos Athanassakis. Baltimore: Johns Hopkins University Press, 2004.

Hobbes, Thomas. *The Elements of Law Natural and Politic: Part 1, Human Nature.* New York: Oxford, 1994 [1640].

——. "Letter of January, 1650 to Robert Payne." In *Hobbes: Une chronique, cheminement de sa penseés et de sa vie,* by Karl Schuhmann, 114–16. Paris: Librairie Philosophique J. Vrin, 1998.

——. *Leviathan.* New York: Cambridge University Press, 1991 [1651].

Hochman, Louis C. "Protest at Morris Knolls HS: Dress Code Promotes 'Rape Culture.'" NJ.com. Last modified June 18, 2014. http://www.nj.com/morris/index.ssf/2014/06/protest_at_morris_knolls_hs_dress_code_promotes_rape_culture.html.

The Holy Bible. New York: Oxford University Press, 1973.

Hom, Sabrina L. "Antigone Falters: Reflections on the Sustainability of Revolutionary Subjects." In *Thinking With Irigaray,* ed. Sabrina L. Hom, Serene Khader, and Mary C. Rawlinson, 247–64. Albany: SUNY Press, 2011.

Honig, Bonnie. *Antigone Interrupted.* Cambridge: Cambridge University Press, 2013.

———. "Ismene's Forced Choice: Sacrifice and Sorority in Sophocles' Antigone." *Arethusa* 44, no. 1 (Winter 2011): 29–68.

Hossain, Emran. "Rana Plaza Collapse Victims Still Waiting for Compensation." *Huffington Post,* August 6, 2013.

Huffer, Lynne. "Foucault's Fossils: The Return to Nature and Life Itself in Anthropocene Feminism." Presentation at Anthropocene Feminism: A Center for Twenty-first-Century Studies conference at the University of Wisconsin-Milwaukee, Milwaukee, Wisconsin, April 10–12, 2014.

International Commission on the Future of Food. "Manifesto on the Future of Seed." In *Manifestos on the Future of Food and Seed,* ed. Vandana Shiva, 76–102. Cambridge: South End, 2007.

"Intimate Partner Violence: Data Sources." *Centers for Disease Control.* Accessed November 3, 2014. http://www.cdc.gov/violenceprevention/intimatepartnerviolence/data sources.html.

Irigaray, Luce. "A Chance for Life." In *Sexes and Genealogies,* 183–206. Trans. Gillian C. Gill. New York: Columbia University Press, 1993.

———. "A Chance to Live." In *Thinking the Difference: For a Peaceful Revolution,* 1–36. Trans. Karin Montin. New York: Routledge, 1994.

———. *Democracy Begins Between Two.* London: Athlone, 2000.

———. "The Eternal Irony of the Community." In *Speculum of the Other Woman,* 214–26. Trans. Gillian C. Gill. Ithaca, NY: Cornell University Press, 1985.

———. *An Ethics of Sexual Difference.* Trans. Carolyn Burke and Gillian C. Gill. Ithaca, NY: Cornell University Press, 1993.

———. "How to Manage the Transition from Natural to Civil Coexistence?" In *Democracy Begins Between Two,* 49–59. London: Athlone, 2000.

———. "Human Nature Is Two." In *I Love to You: Sketch for a Felicity Within History,* 35–42. Trans. Alison Martin. New York: Routledge, 1996.

———. *I Love to You: Sketch for a Felicity Within History.* Trans. Alison Martin. New York: Routledge, 1996.

———. *Je, Tu, Nous: Toward a Culture of Differences.* New York: Routledge, 2007.

———. "The Question of the Other." In *Democracy Begins Between Two,* 121–41. London: Athlone, 2000.

———. *Sexes and Genealogies.* Trans. Gillian C. Gill. New York: Columbia University Press, 1993.

———. *Speculum of the Other Woman.* Trans. Gillian C. Gill. Ithaca, NY: Cornell University Press, 1985.

———. "Ten Suggestions for the Construction of the European Union." In *Democracy Begins Between Two,* 156–64. London: Athlone, 2000.

———. *Thinking the Difference.* Trans. Karin Montin. New York: Routledge, 1994.

———. *This Sex Which Is Not One.* Trans. Carolyn Burke and Catherine Porter. Ithaca, NY: Cornell University Press, 1985.

———. *To Be Two*. Trans. Monique Rhodes and Marco F. Cocito-Monoc. New York: Routledge, 2001.

———. "A Two-Subject Culture." In *Democracy Begins Between Two*, 142–55. London: Athlone, 2000.

Jaggar, Alison. "Global Responsibility and Western Feminism." In *Feminist Interventions in Ethics and Politics: Feminist Ethics and Social Theory*, ed. Barbara S. Andrew, Jean Keller, and Lisa H. Schwartzman, 185–200. Lanham, MD: Rowman and Littlefield, 2005.

James, Henry. *Roderick Random*. New York: Penguin, 1986.

Johnson, Ian. "China's Great Uprooting: Moving 250 Million Into Cities." *New York Times*, June 15, 2013.

Kane, Stefan, and Dominique Martin. "National Self-Sufficiency in Reproductive Resources: An Innovative Response to Transnational Reproductive Travel." *International Journal of Feminist Approaches to Bioethics* 7, no. 2 (Fall 2014): 10–44.

Kant, Immanuel. *Groundwork of the Metaphysic of Morals*. Trans. H. J. Paton. New York: Harper Torchbooks, 1964.

———. "Idea for a Universal History with Cosmopolitan Intent." Trans. Carl J. Friedrich. In *Basic Writings of Kant*, ed. Allen W. Wood, 117–32. New York: Random House, 2001.

———. "To Eternal Peace." Trans. Carl J. Friedrich. In *Basic Writings of Kant*, ed. Allen W. Wood, 433–76. New York: Random House, 2001.

Kantor, Jodi. "Starbucks to Revise Policies to End Irregular Schedules for Its 130,000 Baristas." *New York Times*, August 14, 2014.

———. "Working Anything But 9 to 5." *New York Times*, August 13, 2014.

Keltner, Jane, ed. "The Top 12 Fall Fashion Trends 2009." *Teen Vogue*. Last modified June 2009. http://www.teenvogue.com/fashion/fall-trends/2009-06/fall-fashion-top-12/.

Kemp, Joe. "Iowa Court OKs Firing of Female Dental Assistant for Being 'Too Irresistibly' Attractive." *New York Daily News*, December 22, 2012.

Kerényi, Carl. *Eleusis*. Trans. Ralph Manheim. Princeton: Princeton University Press, 1967.

Khader, Serene J. *Adaptive Preferences and Women's Empowerment*. New York: Oxford University Press, 2011.

Kilbourne, Jean. "Beauty . . . and the Beast of Advertising." *Media and Values* 49 (Winter 1990).

Kittay, Eva Feder. "Equality, Dignity and Disability." In *Perspectives on Equality: The Second Seamus Heaney Lectures*, ed. Mary Ann Lyons and Fionnuala Waldron. Dublin: Liffey, 2005.

———. *Love's Labor: Essays on Women, Equality, and Dependency*. New York: Routledge, 1999.

Kocieniewski, David. "A Shuffle of Aluminum, but to Banks, Pure Gold." *New York Times*, July 20, 2013.

Kolker, Robert. *Lost Girls: An Unsolved American Mystery*. New York: Harper Collins, 2013.

Kristof, Nicholas and Sheryl WuDunn. *Half the Sky: Turning Oppression into Opportunity for Women Worldwide*. New York: Knopf, 2009.

———. *A Path Appears: Transforming Lives, Creating Opportunity*. New York: Knopf, 2014.

Krugman, Paul. "Those Lazy Jobless." *New York Times,* September 22, 2014.

Lang, Tim and Erik Millstone. *The Atlas of Food.* Berkeley: University of California Press, 2008.

Law, Malcolm, and Nicholas Wald. "Why Heart Disease Mortality Is Low in France: The Time Lag Explanation." *British Journal of Medicine* 318, no. 7198 (1999): 1471–1480.

Le Guin, Ursula K. *The Dispossessed.* New York: Harper and Row, 1974.

Leibniz, Gottfried Wilhelm von. *Monadology and Other Philosophical Essays.* Trans. P. and A. M. Schrecker. Indianapolis: Bobbs-Merrill, 1963.

Lerner, Sharon. *The War on Moms: Life in a Family-Unfriendly Nation.* Hoboken, NJ: Wiley, 2010.

Lévi-Strauss, Claude. *The Raw and the Cooked.* New York: Harper and Row, 1969.

Levinas, Emmanuel. *Otherwise Than Being or Beyond Essence.* Trans. Alphonso Lingis. The Hague: Nijhoff, 1981.

Lunt, Neal, Richard Smith, Mark Exworthy, Stephen T. Green, Daniel Horstall, and Russell Mannion. "Medical Tourism. Treatments, Markets, and Health Systems Implications: A Scoping Review." *Organization for Economic Cooperation and Development.* Accessed November 3, 2014. http://www.oecd.org/els/health-systems/internationaltradeinhealth services.htm.

Macklin, Ruth. "Is There Anything Wrong with Surrogate Motherhood? An Ethical Analysis." In *Surrogate Motherhood: Politics and Privacy.* Bloomington: Indiana University Press, 1990.

——. "Reproductive Tourism in India: Is Surrogacy Ethical?" *International Journal of Feminist Approaches to Bioethics Blog,* October 10, 2013. http://www.ijfab.org/blog/reproductive-tourism-in-india-is-surrogacy-ethical/.

Maqbool, Aleem. "Pakistan Rape Victim Mukhtar Mai Faces New Injustice." Last modified April 27, 2011. http://www.bbc.co.uk/news/world-south-asia-13205439.

Marder, Michael. *Plant-Thinking: A Philosophy of Vegetal Life.* New York: Columbia University Press, 2013.

Mason, Jim and Peter Singer. *The Ethics of What We Eat: Why Our Food Choices Matter.* New York: Rodale, 2006.

McMillan, Tracie. *The American Way of Eating: Undercover at Walmart, Applebee's, Farm Fields, and the Dinner Table.* New York: Scribner, 2012.

Melville, Herman. *Moby Dick.* New York: Random House, 1952 [1851].

Mignon, Ernest. *Les mots du general.* Paris: Fayard, 1962.

Mill, John Stuart. *On Liberty.* New York: Oxford University Press, 1991 [1859].

Millennium Ecosystem Assessment. *Ecosystems and Human Well-being.* Washington, DC: Island, 2005.

Mills, Patricia Jagentowicz. "Hegel's *Antigone.*" In *Feminist Interpretations of G. W. F. Hegel,* ed. Patricia Jagentowicz Mills, 59–88. University Park: Pennsylvania State University Press, 1995.

Moisse, Katie. "10-Year-Old Model's Grown-up Look: High Fashion or High Risk?" *ABC News.* Last modified August 4, 2011. http://abcnews.go.com/Health/w_MindBody Resource/10-year-models-grown-high-fashion-high-risk/story?id=14221160.

Monroe, James. "First Inaugural Address." In *A Documentary History of the United States*, ed. Richard D. Heffner. New York: Signet/Mentor, 1965.

"Monsanto 2012 Annual Report." Monsanto. Accessed October 31, 2014. http://www .monsanto.com/global/hu/documents/monsanto-2012-annual-report.pdf.

Montanari, Massimo. *Food Is Culture*. New York: Columbia University Press, 2006.

Moscucci, Ornella. *The Science of Woman: Gynaecology and Gender in England 1800–1929*. Cambridge: Cambridge University Press, 1993.

Narayan, Thelma. "Challenges of the National Rural Health Mission." *Indian Journal of Medical Ethics* 2, no. 2 (2005): 42–43.

Narayan, Uma. "Contesting Cultures: 'Westernization,' Respect for Cultures, and Third-World Feminists." In *Dislocating Cultures: Identities, Traditions, and Third World Feminism*. New York: Routledge, 1997.

New York Times editorial board. "Goldman Sachs Aluminum Pile." *New York Times*, July 26, 2013.

Nestle, Marion. *Food Politics: How the Food Industry Influences Nutrition and Health*. Berkeley: University of California Press, 2002.

Nguyan, Binh T., and Lisa M. Powell. "The Impact of Restaurant Consumption Among U.S. Adults: Effects on Energy and Nutrient Intakes." *Public Health Nutrition* 7, no. 11, 2445–52.

Nonnus. *Dionysiaca*. Trans. W. H. D. Rouse. Oxford: Oxford University Press, 1984.

Nussbaum, Martha C. *Women and Human Development: The Capabilities Approach*. New York: Cambridge University Press, 2000.

Odell, Amy. "Spring 2009's Most Dangerous Shoes." In *The Cut: New York Magazine's Fashion Blog* (October 1, 2008). http://nymag.com/daily/fashion/2008/10/death_shoes .html.

The Odyssey of Homer. Trans. Richmond Lattimore. New York: Harper Colophon, 1967.

O'Neill, June E. and M. Anne Hill. "Civic Report 17: Gaining Ground? Measuring the Impact of Welfare Reform on Welfare and Work." Manhattan Institute for Policy Research. Last modified July 2001. http://www.manhattan-institute.org/html/cr_17.htm.

O'Neill, Onora. Plenary address to the International Association of Bioethics World Congress, Rijeka, Croatia, September 3–4, 2008.

——. "Rights, Obligations, and World Hunger." In *Global Ethics: Seminal Essays,* ed. Thomas Pogge and Keith Horton, 139–156. St. Paul: Paragon House, 2008.

Ovid. *Metamorphoses*. Trans. Frank Justus Miller. Cambridge: Harvard University Press, 1968.

Patel, Raj. *Stuffed and Starved*. Brooklyn, NY: Melville House, 2012.

Paulson, Ken. "Ag-gag Bills Harm Free Speech." *USA Today,* April 17, 2013.

Pausanias. *Description of Greece*. Cambridge: Harvard University Press, 1935.

Pavetti, LaDonna and Liz Schott. "TANF's Inadequate Response to the Recession Highlights Weakness of Block Grant Structure." *Center on Budget and Policy Priorities*. Last modified July 14, 2011. http://www.cbpp.org/cms/?fa=view&id=3534.

Philbrick, Nathaniel. *Mayflower: A Story of Courage, Community, and War.* New York: Penguin, 2006.

Pindar. *Olympian Ode.* Trans. William H. Rice. Cambridge: Harvard University Press, 1997.

Pinkard, Terry. *Hegel's Phenomenology: The Sociality of Reason.* New York: Cambridge, 1996.

Plato. *Republic.* Trans. C. D. C. Reeve. Indianapolis: Hackett, 2004.

Pollan, Michael. *The Omnivore's Dilemma.* New York: Penguin, 2007.

Potter, Van Rensselaer. *Bioethics: Bridge to the Future.* New York: Prentice-Hall, 1971.

Proust, Marcel. *À la recherche du temps perdu.* Paris: Pléiade, 1987.

Ramsey, Paul. *The Patient as Person.* New Haven: Yale University Press, 1974.

Rawlinson, Mary C. "Beyond Virtue and the Law." In *Trauma, Truth, and Reconciliation,* ed. Nancy Nyquist Potter, 139–70. New York: Oxford, 2006.

——. "Foucault's Strategy: Knowledge, Power, and the Specificity of Truth." *Journal of Medicine and Philosophy* 12, no. 4 (November 1987): 371–95.

——. "Obama and Agribusiness." *International Journal of Feminist Approaches to Bioethics Blog,* May 31, 2013. http://www.ijfab.org/blog/obama-and-agribusiness/.

——. "Psychoanalytic Discourse and the Feminine Voice." *Journal of Medicine and Philosophy* 7, no. 2 (May 1982): 153–78.

——. "The Right to Life: Rethinking Universalism in Bioethics." In *Feminist Bioethics: At the Center, on the Margins,* ed. Laurel Baldwin-Ragaven, Petya Fitzpatrick, and Jackie Leach Scully, 107–30. Baltimore: Johns Hopkins University Press, 2010.

——. "Toward an Ethics of Place: A Philosophical Analysis of Cultural Tourism." *International Studies in Philosophy* 38, no. 2 (2007): 141–58.

Reineke, Sandra. "*In vitro veritas*: New Reproductive and Genetic Technologies in Contemporary France." *International Journal of Feminist Approaches to Bioethics* 1, no. 1 (Spring 2008): 91–125.

Rilke, Rainer Maria. *Duino Elegies.* Trans. Stephen Garmey and Jay Wilson. New York: Harper-Colophon, 1972.

Roosevelt, Franklin D. "First Inaugural Address." In *A Documentary History of the United States,* ed. Richard D. Heffner, 274–78. New York: Signet, 1965.

——. "The 'Four Freedoms' Speech." In *A Documentary History of the United States,* ed. Richard D. Heffner, 290–97. New York: Signet, 1965.

Rosenthal, Elizabeth. "American Way of Birth, Costliest in the World." *New York Times,* June 30, 2013.

Rousseau, Jean-Jacques. *Discourse on Inequality.* Trans. Franklin Philip. New York: Oxford University Press, 1994 [1755].

——. *Emile; or, On Education.* Trans. Allan Bloom. New York: Basic Books, 1979 [1762].

——. *Reveries of a Solitary Walker.* Trans. Peter France. New York: Penguin, 1979 [1778].

——. *The Social Contract.* Trans. Maurice Cranston. New York: Penguin, 1988.

Rozin, P., K. Kabnick, E. Pete, C. Fischler, and C. Shields. "The Ecology of Eating: Smaller Portions Sizes in France Than in the United States Helps Explain the French Paradox."

Psychological Science 14, no. 5 (2003): 450–54. http. //www.blackwell-synergy.com/doi/full10.1111/1467-9280.02452.

Rudel, Thomas K., Ruth Defries, Gregory P. Asner, and William F. Laurence. "Changing Drivers of Deforestation and New Opportunities for Conservation." *Conservation Biology* 23, no. 6 (2009): 1396–405.

Russell, Louise B., Martha R. Gold, Joanna E. Siegel, Norman Daniels, and Milton C. Weinstein, "The Role of Cost-Effectiveness Analysis in Health and Medicine." *Journal of the American Medical Association* 276, no. 14 (1996): 1172–77.

Rysst, Mari. "'I Am Only Ten Years Old': Femininities, Clothing-Fashion Codes and the Intergenerational Gap of Interpretation of Young Girls' Clothes." *Childhood* 17, no. 1 (February 2010): 76–93.

Sadikman, Lisa. "A Dress Code of Her Own: Teaching Our Girls Body Confidence." *Huffington Post,* June 10, 2014.

Saltzberg, Elayne A., and Joan C. Chrisler. "Beauty Is the Beast: Psychological Effects of the Pursuit of the Perfect Female Body." In *Women: A Feminist Perspective*, ed. Jo Freeman, 306–15. Mountain View, CA: Mayfield, 1995.

Sartre, Jean-Paul. *Being and Nothingness.* Trans. Hazel E. Barnes. New York: Washington Square, 1993 [1943].

Schatz, J. L. "A War on Freedom and Food." *Warscapes.* Last modified April 24, 2013. http://www.warscapes.com/opinion/war-freedom-and-food.

Sen, Amartya. "The Concept of Development." In *Global Ethics: Seminal Essays*, ed. Keith Horton, and Thomas Pogge, 157–80. St. Paul: Paragon House, 2008.

——. *Development as Freedom.* Oxford: Oxford University Press, 1999.

——. "Women's Agency and Social Change." In *Development as Freedom*, 189–203. New York: Knopf, 1999.

"Several Models Fall During Hervé Léger Show." *Fashion Week News.* Last modified February 17, 2009. http://www.fashionweeknews.com/2009/02/17/several-models-fall-during-herve-leger-show/.

Shiva, Vandana. *Earth Democracy: Justice, Sustainability, and Peace.* Brooklyn, NY: South End, 2005.

——, ed. *Manifestos on the Future of Food and Seed.* Cambridge: South End, 2007.

——. "The Seeds of Suicide: How Monsanto Destroys Farming." Global Research. Last modified March 13, 2014. http://www.globalresearch.ca/the-seeds-of-suicide-how-monsanto-destroys-farming/5329947.

——. *Staying Alive: Women, Ecology, and Development.* Brooklyn, NY: South End, 2010.

——. *Stolen Harvest: The Hijacking of the Global Food Supply.* Brooklyn, NY: South End, 2000.

Sin City. Frank Miller, director. Miramax, 2005.

Singh, Jaswant. "Budget 2003–2004." Presented to Parliament, Delhi, India, February 28, 2003.

Site officiel du musée du Louvre. Accessed October 31, 2014. http://cartelfr.louvre.fr/cartelfr/visite?srv=car_not_frame&idNotice=9294&langue=fr.

Slaughter, Joseph. *Human Rights, Inc.: The World Novel, Narrative Form, and International Law.* New York: Fordham University Press, 2007.

Smith, Peggie R. "Elder Care, Gender, and Work: The Work-Family Issue in the Twenty-first Century." *Berkley Journal of Employment and Labor Law* 25, no. 2 (2004): 351–400.

Smith, William. *A Dictionary of Greek and Roman Antiquities,* vol. 2. London: John Murray, 1891.

Soekirman. "Taking the Indonesian Nutrition History to Leap Into the Betterment of Future Generations: Development of the Indonesian Nutrition Guidelines." *Asia Pacific Journal of Clinical Nutrition* 20, no. 3 (2011): 448.

Sophocles. *Antigone.* Trans. David Grene and Richmond Lattimore. Chicago: University of Chicago Press, 1991.

———. *Antigone.* Trans. F. Storr. Cambridge: Harvard University Press, 1912.

———. *Oedipus at Colonus.* Trans. F. Storr. Cambridge: Harvard University Press, 1912.

Sridhar, V. "Why Do Farmers Commit Suicide? The Case of Andhra Pradesh." *Economic and Political Weekly* 41, no. 16 (2006): 1559–65.

Stein, Haley. "Intellectual Property and Genetically Modified Seeds: The United States, Trade, and the Developing World." *Northwestern Journal of Technology and Intellectual Property* 3, no. 2 (Spring 2005): 160–78.

Steiner, Leslie Morgan. *Mommy Wars.* New York: Random House, 2007.

Stengers, Jean, and Anne van Neck. *Masturbation: The History of a Great Terror.* Trans. Kathryn Hoffman. New York: Palgrave Macmillan, 2001.

Swinburn, Boyd A., Gary Sacks, Kevin D. Hall, Klim McPherson, Diane T. Finegood, and Marjory L. Moody. "The Global Obesity Pandemic: Shaped by Global Drivers and Local Environments." *Lancet* 37, no. 9793 (2011): 804–14.

"Takeout Foods, Restaurant Meals Tied to Obesity Trend." *University of Rochester Medical Center Health Encyclopedia Online,* January 11, 2015.

Turner, Leigh. "Global Health Inequalities and Bioethics." In *The Ethics of Bioethics: Mapping the Moral Landscape,* ed. Lisa A. Eckenwiler and Felicia G. Cohn, 229–40. Baltimore: Johns Hopkins University Press, 2007.

United Nations Educational, Scientific and Cultural Organization. "Bioethics." UNESCO.org. Accessed May 15, 2014. http://www.unesco.org/new/en/social-and-human-sciences/themes/bioethics/.

———. "Universal Declaration on Bioethics and Human Rights." UNESCO.org. Last modified October 19, 2005. http://www.unesco.org/new/en/social-and-human-sciences/themes/bioethics/bioethics-and-human-rights/.

United Nations Economic and Social Commission for Asia and the Pacific. "Report of the Regional Implementation Meeting for Asia and the Pacific for the Sixteenth Session of the Commission on Sustainable Development." Sustainable Development Knowledge Platform. Last modified November 27, 2007. http://sustainabledevelopment.un.org/content/documents/escap_doc.pdf.

United Nations Industrial Development Organization. "Agribusiness Development: Transforming Rural Life to Create Wealth." Last modified 2013. http://www.unido

.org/fileadmin/user_media_upgrade/What_we_do/Topics/Agribusiness_and_rural/
UNIDO_Agribusiness_development.pdf.

———. "Fighting Poverty by Fostering Agro-value Chains." *Agribusiness Development:
Transforming Rural Life to Create Wealth.* 2012.

United Nations Millennium Ecosystem Assessment. 2005. http://www.millenniumassess
ment.org/en/About.html.

United Nations Office on Drugs and Crime (UNODC). "Global Report on Trafficking
in Persons." Last modified February 2009. http://www.unodc.org/documents/Global
_Report_on_TIP.pdf.

United States Agency for International Development. "New Alliance for Food Security
and Nutrition." USAID. Last modified May 31, 2013. http://www.usaid.gov/unga/
new-alliance.

Urbina, Ian. "Buying Overseas Clothing, U.S. Flouts Its Own Advice." *New York Times,* December 23, 2013.

U.S. Department of Justice, Bureau of Justice Statistics. *Black Victims of Violent Crime*, by Er-
ika Harrell. August 2007, NCJ 214258. http://www.bjs.gov/content/pub/pdf/bvvc.pdf.

"La Via Campesina: International Peasant Movement." *La Via Campesina.* Accessed October 31, 2014. http://viacampesina.org/en/.

Warner, Judith. "Outsourced Wombs." *New York Times,* January 3, 2008.

Weiss-Wolf, Jennifer. "My Daughter Was Dress-Coded for Wearing Shorts." *Slate.* Last
modified June 9, 2014. http://www.slate.com/blogs/xx_factor/2014/06/09/dress
_codes_and_the_fingertip_rule_schools_should_not_be_telling_girls_that.html.

White, Scott F., et al. "Gender-Related Differences in the Pathways to and Characteristics of
U.S. Medical School Deanships." *Academic Medicine* 87, no. 8 (2012): 1015–23.

"Why Does Monsanto Sue Farmers Who Save Seeds?" Monsanto. Accessed October 31,
2014. http://www.monsanto.com/newsviews.

Willett, Cynthia. *Interspecies Ethics.* New York: Columbia University Press, 2014.

Winckelmann, Johann Joachim. "Drapery." In *The History of Ancient Art,* vol. 4. Trans.
G. Henry Lodge. Boston: James R. Osgood, 1872.

———. *The History of Ancient Art.* Trans. G. Henry Lodge. Boston: James R. Osgood, 1872.

Winnicott, D. W. *Playing and Reality.* London: Routledge, 1991.

Wolff, E. N. "The Asset Price Meltdown and the Wealth of the Middle Class." US2010 Project. Providence, RI: Brown University, 2012. http://www.s4.brown.edu/us2010/Data/
Report/report05012013.pdf.

Wolfson, Julia A., and Sara N. Bleich. "Is Cooking at Home Associated with Better Diet
Quality or Weight-Loss Intention?" *Public Health Nutrition,* published online November 17, 2014, DOI: http://dx.doi.org/10.1017/S1368980014001943.

Wollstonecraft, Mary. *A Vindication of the Rights of Woman.* New York: Oxford University
Press, 1994.

"Women's Clothing Stores in the U.S.: Market Research Report." *IbisWorld.* Accessed
June 30, 2014.

Woodiwiss, Anthony. *Human Rights.* Oxford: Routledge, 2005.

World Bank. *Agriculture for Development: World Development Report, 2008.* Washington, DC: International Bank for Reconstruction and Development/World Bank, 2007.

———. "World Bank Group Agriculture Action Plan, 2010–12." Last modified July 2009. http://siteresources.worldbank.org/INTARD/Resources/Agriculture_Action_Plan _web.pdf.

World Health Organization. "Obesity and Overweight: Fact Sheet No. 311." World Health Organization. Last modified August 2014. http://www.who.int/mediacentre/ factsheets/fs311/en/.

Index

GPSR Authorized Representative: Easy Access System Europe, Mustamäe tee
50, 10621 Tallinn, Estonia, gpsr.requests@easproject.com

www.ingramcontent.com/pod-product-compliance
Lightning Source LLC
Chambersburg PA
CBHW060029030426
42334CB00019B/2237